Healthy Dining

in Orange County

Third Edition

Restaurant Nutrition Guide

Featuring Healthy Entrees from
86 Popular Orange County Restaurants

Including:

✓✓ **Calories**   ✓✓ **Cholesterol**
✓✓ **Fat**   ✓✓ **Sodium**

Diabetic Food Exchanges and Other Information

by

Accents On Health, Inc.

Authors: Anita Jones, M.P.H.
              Esther Hill, Ph.D.
              Erica Bohm, M.S.

Healthy Dining
in Orange County
Third Edition

Restaurant Nutrition Guide

by

Accents On Health, Inc.

Authors:

Anita Jones, M.P.H., Esther Hill, Ph.D., and Erica Bohm, M.S.

Restaurant and Nutrition Information:

Accents On Health, Inc., 4945 Mercury St., San Diego, CA 92111
(619) 541-2049

Book Publication and Sales:

Hill & Hill Publishing, P.O. Box 927215, San Diego, CA 92192-7215
(619) 453-3814 or (800) 953-DINE

Graphics by Patricia Mattison and Ramon Hutson
Photos by Rachael Kutras (619) 558-7238

Library of Congress Cataloging in Publication Data
Jones, Anita
Healthy Dining in Orange County
1, Nutrition. 2, Diet. 3, Restaurant Food,
I. Title   II. Hill, Esther   III. Bohm, Erica
91-71724
ISBN 1-879754-12-6

Table of Contents

About *Healthy Dining* and Accents On Health

Healthy Dining's team of highly qualified nutrition and health professionals is committed to an ambitious and exciting vision: to foster an ever-expanding trend toward healthier restaurant selections. The *Healthy Dining* project began in San Diego in 1990 and expanded to Orange County and Los Angeles. The team has worked with hundreds of restaurants throughout Southern California and has analyzed over 4,000 menu items for nutrition content.

Healthy Dining is earning respect from all corners -- health professionals, the media, the restaurant industry, and tens of thousands of consumers, many of whom write and call, expressing appreciation for the impact that *Healthy Dining* continues to make in Southern California. The *Healthy Dining* program is a joint venture between Hill & Hill Publishing and Accents On Health, Inc., a health and wellness organization based in San Diego.

About the *Healthy Dining in Orange County* Team:

Anita Jones, M.P.H. -- Author and Director

Anita Jones earned her Master's Degree in Public Health from San Diego State University. Her background includes extensive work in the health and nutrition fields, both with individuals and with community group education and support sessions. Anita is one of the founders of the *Healthy Dining* program and the primary author of the book. She has directed the *Healthy Dining* project from its inception to a growing community program. She also oversees the nutrition analysis and directs public relations and promotion.

Erica Bohm, M.S. -- Co-author and Regional Director

Erica Bohm earned her Master's Degree in Community Health Sciences from New York City's Hunter College. Her experience includes nutrition education, cholesterol reduction, weight control and smoking cessation. During her 18 years in the health field, Erica has worked for the American Red Cross, the American Health Foundation, and other health organizations, research projects and businesses. Her roles in *Healthy Dining* include seminar presentations, program promotion, and networking with restaurants, health professionals, community organizations, and the media.

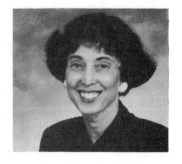

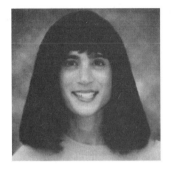

Susan Goldstein -- Orange County Regional Director

Susan Goldstein earned her degree in Human Development and Family Studies from Cornell University. She has a diverse background with experience in corporate business and voluntary health organizations. Susan works directly with the *Healthy Dining* restaurants to implement the program with owners, managers and chefs. She also promotes *Healthy Dining* in the county through special events, marketing, community relations, contacts with health organizations, and publicity.

Esther Hill, Ph.D. -- Editor/Publisher

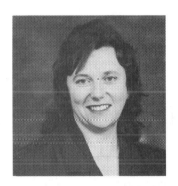

Esther Hill, a physiologist with a Ph.D. in Biomathematics, worked for over 15 years in medical research at the University of California at San Diego and published over 30 scientific articles. Her motivation for being involved in this project comes largely from dealing with her son's unstable diabetes. Dr. Hill's family has found traveling and restaurant dining difficult, and she understands why nutrition information is so important to those with dietary restrictions. Dr. Hill is one of the founders of the *Healthy Dining* program, and directs typesetting, editing and publishing.

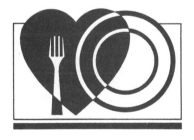

For More Information:

For information on nutrition analysis and special events (speakers, health fairs, tastings, and cooking demonstrations for business or the community), please call Accents On Health:

(619) 541-2049 or (800) 266-2049.

To order books by mail, or for information on wholesale prices or using the book as a fund-raiser, please call Hill & Hill Publishing:

(619) 453-3814 or (800) 953-DINE.

Acknowledgements

Cindy Maynard, R.D., M.S. serves as a consulting dietitian for *Healthy Dining*. She works at Mesa Vista Hospital in San Diego and also has her own private practice, specializing in nutrition counseling, sports nutrition and eating disorders.

Mary Ellen Mann has worked with *Healthy Dining* in contacting various health professionals and organizations in the area and handling correspondence. We thank her for her contributions.

We also extend our sincerest appreciation to the following respected professionals who reviewed this book:

John Campbell, M.D., Pathologist
Charlotte Crucean, Ph.D., Clinical Psychologist
Marci Daniels, J.D.
Mila De Los Reyes, M.A., R.D., Clinical Nutritionist, Mercy Hospital & Medical Center
Mary Donkersloot, R.D., Private Nutrition Counselor for Personal Nutrition Management
     and author of "Fast Food Diet: Quick & Healthy Eating at Home and on the Go"
Michele Edwards, Assist. Dir. Public Education, Am. Cancer Society, San Diego Unit
Therese A. Eyre, M.S., R.D., Obesity Treatment Team Manager, Tri-City Medical Center
     and Past President of the San Diego Dietetics Association
Betsy Horton-La Forge, R.D., M.P.H., Director of Wellness Center, Grossmont Hospital
Anita Johnson, M.S., UCSD Cancer Center
Jeanne Jones, Author of 20 cookbooks and internationally syndicated columnist
Dale Kooistra, M.D.
Ralph La Forge, Director of Health Promotion, San Diego Cardiac Center Medical Group
Cindy Maynard, M.S., R.D., Chief Clinical Dietitian, Mesa Vista Hospital
Margaret Miller, R.D., Scripps Clinic and Research Foundation
Wayne I. Newton, M.D., Cardiovascular Surgeon
Susan Plese, Marketing and Communications
Patricia Porter, Cardiopulmonary Technologist
Susan Slaughter, Jazzercise and "Know More Diet" Instructor
Cindy Stack-Keer, R.D., Health Education, Kaiser Permanente
Jamie Steele, President of Fitness West, Inc., Steele Bodies, Island Fitness
Patti Tveit-Milligan, M.S., R.D.
Suzanne Weeks, R.D., Consulting Nutritionist, Scripps Center for Executive Health
Margaret Wing-Peterson, M.S., R.D., Dietitian for San Diego Cardiac Center

And finally, we especially thank the participating restaurants for the effort they put into preparing this information -- and all health-conscious diners who are supporting *Healthy Dining*. Thanks for your enthusiasm and best wishes for a healthy year of dining out!

Foreword

The surprising truth about dining out

You think you are health conscious. You pick chicken or fish from restaurant menus and believe you'll be safe by doing so. Read on!

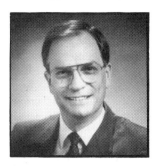

Accents On Health has analyzed thousands of restaurant recipes and found lots of surprises. Menu descriptions just aren't enough, and you rarely know what you're getting!

But now you can be sure. The menus that appear within these pages have passed the closest scrutiny. You'll find great tasting food here that's also good for you! As you can see, these participating restaurants have demonstrated their interest in your health.

You, who are watching your diet, counting calories, and eating less cholesterol -- you win! If you have a heart problem and severe restrictions -- you can dine out too. Watching your sodium (salt)? -- come along! Even those with diabetes can safely leave home and venture into the wonderful, romantic world of dining out, because diabetic food exchange values are printed with every menu entree.

Hooray for the restaurants that are making this possible, and for everyone who is health conscious -- all of you! The information you need is here. Read this guide to the restaurants that proudly display their nutrition information in the *Healthy Dining* menus. Pick a restaurant from this book, not by chance!

David G. Daniels, M.D.

P.S. Please tell everyone in your restaurant -- the manager, the hostess, the waiting staff -- tell everyone why you are there. Your business and your requests for *Healthy Dining* menus are the strongest motivations for them to continue with the *Healthy Dining* program. They need to hear from you, their customers, that it was worthwhile. So...

> Please ask for *Healthy Dining* menus in the restaurants and
> let them know that you appreciate the healthy menu choices.

Orange County's
Healthy Dining Restaurants

Disclaimer:

The purpose of this book is to provide nutrition information for selected menu items from restaurants that have chosen to participate in the *Healthy Dining* program. Please note that the items listed in this book are not necessarily appropriate or healthy for all individuals. Some people need to be more careful about certain items such as salt or sugar, or have food allergies which put additional restrictions on their food choices. Each individual is responsible, in cooperation with his or her physician, dietitian or other health consultant, for making personal dietary decisions.

Please note that we have not included all the restaurants that serve healthy food, nor are we recommending all entrees from restaurants that are included in this book.

It is also important to note that the numerical values for the nutrition information included in this book are approximations only, and that the categories "Very Low" and "Low" are a better indication of the nutrition content of the menu items.

The nutrition information provided is based on the United States Department of Agriculture (USDA) nutrition information database, the source most commonly used for estimating nutritional content of foods. Participating restaurants supplied their recipes for the computerized analysis. The analyses were completed using the Nutritionist IV Computer program developed by N-Squared Computing in Oregon. Research shows the Nutritionist program to be one of the most current and reliable nutrition analysis programs available. If values for recipe ingredients were not available from the USDA data base, the manufacturer was contacted for the nutrition information. If the manufacturer did not have nutrition information, ingredients were closely matched to a similar product's nutrition information. Data were rounded to the nearest whole number and nearest 1/4 for diabetic exchanges.

All information contained in this book has been carefully compiled and reviewed by qualified health professionals. Nutrition information is based on recipes supplied by the restaurants. Participating restaurants have agreed to prepare food according to the recipes submitted for a period of one year, or to clearly notify customers otherwise.

The authors are not responsible for maintaining quality control over the food that is prepared by the restaurants. The restaurants are ultimately responsible for the quality of the food they serve.

A Fund-Raiser with Good Taste!

Looking for an exciting, effective and innovative way to raise funds for your organization?

Healthy Dining in Orange County is your answer.

Healthy Dining is a great way to raise money:

- unique, attractive, trend-setting book
- distinguishes your group from others selling the "usual" products
- high monetary return to your organization
- priced right
- easy to sell, especially with the valuable restaurant coupons
- informative and useful, with genuine health/educational value
- great gift idea
- can be sold throughout the year
- wide appeal for anyone who:
    - is slimming down
    - leads an active, healthy lifestyle
    - has high cholesterol, high blood pressure, etc.
    - enjoys dining out!

For more information, please contact
Healthy Dining at **(619) 453-3814**

People are talking about *Healthy Dining*...

"Healthy Dining...is a 'nutrition label' for restaurant meals.
This illuminating book provides clear, straightforward information that lets
you enjoy dining out without excess fat, calories, cholesterol and sodium."
- Art Ulene, M.D., Medical Expert on TODAY on NBC

"A road map gets you where you want to go when you travel.
Healthy Dining does the same thing when you dine
out and do not want to do yourself in."
- Annette Globits, R.D., Nutritional education & counseling

"Healthy Dining makes it so easy to achieve and maintain a healthy diet. It's the only
reliable source available that spells out nutritious *and* delicious restaurant choices.
My clients love it. And the book pays for itself with the restaurant coupons!"
- Miriam Matulich, R.D., Hoag Memorial Hospital Presbyterian

"The American Heart Association applauds the participating
restaurants for accommodating the customer of the 90's,
the customer that cares about good health."
- Patricia Lozada-Santone, M.P.H., American Heart Association volunteer

"Reality is...<u>Dining out</u> is part of most lifestyles! In my practice, I teach my
clients how to make practical and realistic dining decisions. *Healthy Dining*
is an excellent tool which helps my clients reach their health and fitness goals."
- Scott Poulalion, R.D., The Sports Club/Irvine

"I always applaud any effort to bring nutritional information to the
community. You've done an outstanding job."
- Jeanne Jones, cookbook author and internationally syndicated columnist

"Healthy Dining makes healthy low-calorie restaurant dining easy.
It's a wonderful tool that allows people the freedom and
enjoyment of restaurant dining without guilt and anxiety."
- Linda Trozzolino, Ph.D., writer and director of weight control programs

"I like KNOWING what I'm eating rather than guessing. The 'Special Requests'
in the book are excellent suggestions -- I order them almost all the time!"
- Jane, Program Coordinator, American Cancer Society

People are talking about *Healthy Dining*...

"We've received a tremendous response to *Healthy Dining*...
The combination of great Orange County restaurants and a book that
fits in so well to today's desire for healthy eating is perfect!"
- Lorna Harris, Promotions Director, KEZY Radio

"I didn't realize until I read this book that I <u>have</u> been avoiding
eating in restaurants in an effort to stay healthy and slim.
Armed with this book, I'm eager to dine out again!"
- Michele Edwards

"Having eaten at many of the restaurants listed, I was delighted to find detailed information...
that will enable me to continue enjoying 'fine dining' and not sacrifice my health!"
- Renee LaBriola, M.A., R.D., Kaiser Permanente

"I have searched far and wide for a restaurant guide that finds
not only good food, but delicious HEALTHY food. My prayers
have been answered with the *Healthy Dining* series!"
- Victor Ettinger, M.D., Medical Director, Bone Diagnostic & Treatment Centres

"Many of the men and women coming through our Corporate Health Services have...positions
[that] demand that they dine out often. *Healthy Dining*...is just the tool we have been
looking for to assist our busy clients in achieving their health and fitness goals."
- James E. McGinley, UCI Corporate Health Services

"*Healthy Dining* is an invaluable book for those concerned about their health."
- Elmer Dills, KABC Talk Radio

"A fantastic reference for both health educators and their students.
It's like having your own personal dietitian with you while dining out."
- Robert Abelson, Ph.D., Cert. Health & Fitness Instr. and UCLA Extension Health Instructor

"The *Healthy Dining* book is a great addition to our Fat Loss Program -- the members
love it and the book helps our members get true results and maintain them."
- April Morgan, Fitness & Aerobics Director, The Sports Club Company

"The format of the book makes it easy to access information in a hurry.
I've bought the books for my friends, and I carry it in my car at all times!!!"
- Nancy McNash, Costa Mesa

An Important Message from the *Healthy Dining* Team

Welcome to the **Healthy Dining** "family." This program has grown from San Diego to Orange County to Los Angeles. More than 1000 individuals have participated in this effort, including restaurant chefs and management, health professionals, and members of community organizations. You, the **Healthy Dining** reader and restaurant diner, play an essential role in this as well.

Why? Because restaurants respond to their customers. They need to hear from you that health-conscious menu items and nutrition information are important to you.

Please Help! Here's how you can help **Healthy Dining** to grow in your community:

1. Dine at the restaurants listed in the book, and tell the restaurant staff and/or owners that you appreciate and value their participation in **Healthy Dining**. Also, request the **Healthy Dining** menus at participating restaurants and use the discount coupons.

2. Tell friends, family and business associates about **Healthy Dining**.

3. Tell other restaurants about **Healthy Dining** and recommend that they participate next year.

4. Give **Healthy Dining** books as gifts for birthdays, holidays, etc.

5. Use **Healthy Dining** as a fund-raiser (see page xi).

6. Use **Healthy Dining** restaurants for your catering and party needs.

7. Please call us with your suggestions and feedback (619) 453-3814.

Thanks! We appreciate your support.

How to Use This Book

This introduction summarizes how to interpret the nutrition information for the restaurant menu items. Part I of the book provides more in-depth information to help you become better informed about health and restaurant dining. Part II features nutrition profiles of specific entrees from 86 restaurants at over 425 locations in Orange County.

The Check Mark System - An easy way to find entrees to fit your goals

First, we should define "healthy entree." In this book, a healthy entree is one with high-quality, nutritious calories. In general, these are low or very low in fat, cholesterol, calories and sodium. Because many entrees are not low in all areas, the check mark system will help you easily and quickly identify which entrees best fit your individual dietary goals.

Nutritional guidelines are difficult to set. Each individual has different nutritional needs, and we recognize that. For example, caloric needs vary according to age, gender, activity level, body weight and health goals (e.g., reducing body fat, lowering cholesterol, etc.). Nevertheless, we've provided some general guidelines to make the menu information easy to interpret. These guidelines are based on recommendations by the Surgeon General's Office and the American Heart Association. Details about how the values were chosen are included in Chapters 3 through 6, but here's a quick summary of the check mark meanings:

ENTREE GUIDELINES

Calories	✓✓	Very Low = 0 to 350 calories/entree
	✓	Low = 350 to 600 calories/entree
Fat	✓✓	Very Low = 0 to 10 grams (g)/entree
	✓	Low = 10 to 20 grams (g)/entree
Cholesterol	✓✓	Very Low = 0 to 75 milligrams (mg)/entree
	✓	Low = 75 to 150 milligrams (mg)/entree
Sodium	✓✓	Very Low = 0 to 300 milligrams (mg)/entree
	✓	Low = 300 to 600 milligrams (mg)/entree

It's important to note...

Although the "Low" and "Very Low" designations may not be as strict as some would like to see, they represent fairly high standards for restaurant entrees and are realistic goals for most diners. We've developed an easy-to-read format that will meet most people's needs rather than including very extensive nutrition information that may be necessary for some individuals.

We occasionally include a menu item that is described as "moderate" in one of the nutrient categories. "Moderate" means that the item does not meet the guidelines for "low," but it is less than twice the cut-off value for "low." Some items are listed as "high" in sodium (meaning above 1000 mg. sodium per entree) and are **not** recommended for those watching sodium intake.

Please note that these are general guidelines developed for the general public. You, your physician and your dietitian are responsible for setting individual nutritional guidelines, according to your particular health needs.

Depending on your particular dietary goals...

If you are health-conscious and looking for better ways to eat and enhance your overall health, this book will provide an easy way to choose entrees that don't have the hidden calories, fat, cholesterol and sodium you'd rather avoid.

If you want to lose weight, take special note of the calorie and fat categories and choose items that are very low (✓✓) or low (✓) in these areas (see Chapters 3 and 4).

If you want to reduce your blood cholesterol level, look for items that are very low (✓✓) or low (✓) in both cholesterol and fat (see Chapter 5).

To reduce dietary sodium, select items that are very low (✓✓) or low (✓) in sodium, and request no added salt (see Chapter 6).

If you have diabetes, the "Exchanges" (i.e., Diabetic Exchanges used by the American Diabetes Association) are particularly useful. For more details, see Chapter 7.

If your physician or dietitian has given you daily limits in terms of sodium, cholesterol, etc., by all means note the numerical values as well as the check marks, and be sure they fit your restrictions. You may need to ask for additional modifications to your meal.

We've included brief entree descriptions, but they are not complete ingredient lists. Therefore, if you have food allergies or sensitivities, be sure to emphasize this to the restaurant personnel so they will understand how important it is to prepare your meal according to your specifications.

Comments about serving sizes, dressings and sauces, and side dishes

Remember that the nutrition information published in this book is based on the FULL SERVING (unless stated otherwise). If you eat only 2/3 of the entree, you're only consuming 2/3 of the calories, fat, cholesterol, sodium, etc. So if you're craving an item that is a little higher in a particular area, order it, eat only part, and save the rest for tomorrow.

In some cases the nutrition analysis includes dressings or sauces, and in other cases it does not. We generally recommend that you order sauces and dressings on the side and use them sparingly. Dressings and sauces usually contain 5 to 10 grams of fat (45 to 90 calories) per tablespoon. Depending on your goals, you may choose to completely avoid them, or order them on the side and limit the amount you use. You will likely be served more than one tablespoon, so don't assume you can pour it all on your meal. You can measure out the amount you want using your teaspoon, keeping in mind that 3 teaspoons is equivalent to one tablespoon (Tbs) or ½ ounce (oz).

The check mark system and guidelines listed on the previous page apply to main entrees only. We also feature some side dishes, appetizers, and desserts, and have set the guidelines for calories, fat, cholesterol and sodium equal to 1/3 of the entree guidelines. Other items such as breads are not generally shown because the nutrition values are fairly standard.

GUIDELINES for SIDE DISHES and APPETIZERS†

Calories	✓✓	Very Low = 0 to 117 calories/serving
	✓	Low = 117 to 200 calories/serving
Fat	✓✓	Very Low = 0 to 3 grams (g)/serving
	✓	Low = 3 to 7 grams (g)/serving
Cholesterol	✓✓	Very Low = 0 to 25 milligrams (mg)/serving
	✓	Low = 25 to 50 milligrams (mg)/serving
Sodium	✓✓	Very Low = 0 to 100 milligrams (mg)/serving
	✓	Low = 100 to 200 milligrams (mg)/serving

FOOTNOTES - Summary of what they mean

† Side dish guidelines are 1/3 of entree guidelines
* Primarily unsaturated fat (see Chapter 4)
** If you request no added salt (see Chapter 6)

PRICE RANGE SYMBOL

At the end of each restaurant's introductory paragraph, a price range symbol appears:

$ Average entree under $10
$$ Average entree $10 - $20
$$$ Average entree over $20

How were restaurants selected to be included in this book?

Our goal was to include a wide variety of restaurants. We did not just look for restaurants that specialize in serving "health food," but for a selection of popular restaurants that have a sincere interest in providing healthy foods and nutrition information. If you want organic and natural foods, we have included restaurants that cater to those preferences as well. Vegetarian dishes are available at many of the restaurants. A good clue for vegetarian dishes is to look for items with no cholesterol (no animal products) or very low values, which may indicate small quantities of cheese or dairy products. You may, of course, double check with the restaurant personnel before ordering.

Restaurants participating in this book have a genuine interest in offering healthy choices. They paid a fee for the nutritional analysis, and they have signed an agreement with Accents On Health to prepare the selected entrees in accordance with the recipes they submitted or clearly notify customers otherwise. We highly respect the restaurants included in this book for their interest and commitment to serving healthy entrees. We purposely included many different types of cuisines with a wide range of prices and feel this will have the greatest impact in encouraging all restaurants to offer healthy, delicious choices.

How were entrees selected?

When a restaurant agreed to participate in the *Healthy Dining* Program, our staff of qualified health professionals worked with the chef to select recipes low in fat, cholesterol, calories and sodium.

Our first choice was to find items already on the menu, without making any modifications. This would be the easiest for you and for the restaurant. However, in some cases the recipe analysis didn't meet the *Healthy Dining* guidelines. So we worked with the chef to develop a "Special Request" version which contains less calories, fat, cholesterol and/or sodium than the original dish (see Chapter 2). The analyses listed in this book for the "Special Request" items correspond to the lower calorie, fat, etc. content that you will be served <u>if and only if you make the "Special Request."</u> Otherwise you will be served a meal with considerably higher fat and higher calorie values. See Chapter 2 for examples.

We need your help!

The restaurants in this book have devoted time, money and effort to participate. In many cases the restaurants have modified recipes to meet your needs. Now they need to hear from you that this nutrition information is important to you and that you appreciate their participation in *Healthy Dining*.

> We have provided *Healthy Dining* menus for customers' use at each of the participating restaurants. Please ask for them!

We encourage all the restaurants to pass out *Healthy Dining* menus along with their regular menus. These *Healthy Dining* menus are condensed versions of the book pages. Some restaurants, however, do not automatically provide them -- *you must request the Healthy Dining menus*. And please do! The more that restaurants hear customers asking for specific nutrition information and ordering "Special Requests," the more they will recognize how important healthy dining is to many people.

So if this information is important to you, if you want to have the choice to "order healthy," **PLEASE tell the *Healthy Dining* restaurants**! Please tell other restaurants that you'd like them to participate. This will enable us to include more restaurants and an even greater variety of healthy choices in the next edition of *Healthy Dining in Orange County*.

We welcome your ideas

This program is still growing, and we welcome your ideas on how we can enhance it. Please feel free to write to us with your comments. We update this publication periodically with more restaurants, more healthy entrees, and more nutrition information.

Don't forget to use the valuable restaurant coupons in the back of the book when visiting *Healthy Dining* restaurants!

Part I

Healthy Dining Tips:

Realistic Guidelines and Practical Information

"If you don't smoke, what you eat may be the biggest factor influencing your health."

- U.S. Surgeon General

CHAPTER 1

Health, Lifestyle, Diet, Misconceptions & ... Dining Out

In 1988, the Surgeon General made a startling announcement to the American public:

"If you don't smoke, what you eat may be
the biggest factor influencing your health."

We've come a long way...

Diet has always strongly influenced health and disease. Until the early decades of this century, our country suffered from problems of _undernutrition_. Rickets, pellagra, scurvy, beriberi and goiter plagued our nation. Fortunately, in the United States, the advances in medicine, fortification of foods, and successful cures virtually eliminated the vicious diseases caused by a lack of essential nutrients.

Currently, we've reached a whole new perspective on health and disease. A large body of medical research shows that lifestyle greatly influences health status. It is well recognized that daily health habits -- what we eat and drink, whether or not we smoke, how much exercise we get and how effectively we manage stress -- contribute to _how long and how well_ we live.

The 1988 Surgeon General's Report on Nutrition and Health outlines the substantial impact of dietary practices on health. Five of the ten leading causes of death (heart disease, cancer, stroke, diabetes, and atherosclerosis), which together account for over 2/3 of all deaths in the U.S., are directly related to diet. The report's main conclusion is:

"_Overconsumption_ of certain dietary components is now a major concern for Americans. While many food factors are involved, chief among them is the disproportionate consumption of foods high in fats, often at the expense of foods high in complex carbohydrates and fiber that may be more conducive to health."

-- 1988 Surgeon General's Report on Nutrition and Health --

Clearly, a priority for Americans is to reduce intake of total fat, especially saturated fat, because of the relationship between excess dietary fat and the development of many leading chronic disease conditions.

Dietary guidelines for Americans:

Based on extensive scientific evidence, the following recommendations were developed by the Surgeon General's Office and the American Heart Association:

1. Reduce overall consumption of fat, especially saturated fat. The American Heart Association recommends that no more than 30% of total calories come from fat (the average American diet contains approximately 35% fat). Saturated fat should comprise no more than 10% of the daily diet. Choose foods low in fat such as vegetables, fruits, whole grain foods, fish, lean meats and non-fat dairy products. Use food preparation methods that add little or no fat.

2. Reduce cholesterol consumption to under 300 mg. per day, as recommended by the American Heart Association. The average American consumes about 400 - 600 mg. daily.

3. Reduce intake of sodium by choosing foods relatively low in sodium and limiting the amount of salt in food preparation and at the table. The American Heart Association recommends fewer than 3,000 mg. per day. The average American consumes about 4,000 - 6,000 mg. daily.

4. Achieve and maintain a desirable body weight. To do so, choose a balanced diet in which energy (caloric) intake is consistent with energy expenditure. To reduce caloric intake, limit consumption of foods relatively high in calories, fat, and sugar, and minimize alcohol consumption. Increase energy expenditure through regular exercise.

5. Increase consumption of complex carbohydrates and fiber, such as whole grain foods, cereals, vegetables, fruits, dried beans, peas, and lentils.

Americans are catching on!

We're watching what we eat. Learning more about what we eat. Making healthier choices. We're beginning to cherish our health for its influence on all other aspects of our lives. For top performance, we're eating more high-quality fuel -- more fruits, vegetables and whole grains -- and less beef, butter, whole milk and other foods high in saturated fat.

Since the mid-1970s, consumption of saturated fats has decreased significantly. In addition, U.S. death rates from heart disease have fallen dramatically, close to 25 percent in the last decade. Leading health organizations attribute some of this decline to better medical care but give most of the credit to healthier diets and lifestyles.

Food manufacturers are catching on, but...

Marketing efforts toward our increasingly health-conscious society have intensified in the past several years. Close to 30% of food advertising includes some type of health message. Although this spiraling emphasis on healthy eating from food makers is encouraging, it can be very misleading. Milk flaunts a 2% fat label (meaning 2% of the milk's <u>weight</u> is fat), but 35% of total <u>calories</u> come from fat. Similarly, lunchmeats brag about a 96% lean composition. Again, this means that only 4% of the meat's <u>weight</u> is fat, not 4% of the calories (a high percentage of the weight is water, thus decreasing the percentage weight from fat). Cookies, crackers and chips leap out from shelves with bright "NO CHOLESTEROL" banners, although the amount of total fat or saturated fat seems to be of little concern (at least to the manufacturer). Recently fat-free and cholesterol-free cakes and cookies made their debut into society -- with so much sugar, there's not much room for fat and cholesterol.

Reading between the lines

Until recently, deciphering food labels was a difficult task. Nutrition information on labels was often misleading, confusing and incomplete. Terms such as "low-fat," "light," "natural," and "healthy" had virtually no standardized meaning and could be added to any package, regardless of contents.

Fortunately, since May 1994, the Food and Drug Administration (FDA) has required almost all food packages to display a universal nutrition information label. These new labels are designed to help you easily identify important nutrition information. The FDA has also developed strict guidelines for several nutritional claims commonly used by food manufacturers. For example, any food package stating the product is "low-fat" must now have less than 3 grams of fat per serving. A "low-calorie" food must now contain less than 40 calories per serving. A food package promoting the product as "light" (e.g., light mayonnaise) must now contain 50% less fat or one-third fewer calories than the food with which it is being compared (e.g., regular mayonnaise). If the original product contains more than 50% calories from fat, the fat must be reduced by at least 50% in the "light" product.

Please note that the guidelines set by the FDA for food packages are significantly different from the *Healthy Dining* guidelines because the *Healthy Dining* guidelines represent the better part of a full meal, whereas the FDA guidelines are designed for a single product or serving.

A crusader for healthier fast foods

In April 1990, Phil Sokolof and his non-profit organization, The National Heart Savers Association, attacked American fast food restaurants with full-page ads in large newspapers accusing them of "poisoning" Americans with foods high in saturated fat. A Gallup poll showed that almost 40% of those that saw the ads immediately decreased their visits to fast food restaurants. Just three weeks later, McDonald's responded by removing beef tallow from their French fries. Other fast food chains quickly followed. Sokolof points out that his major goal was to stop fast food from being a *"fast track to a heart attack."*

With Sokolof paving the way, consumers began demanding to know -- just what are we getting in fast food meals? In response, several fast food restaurants now provide nutrition information for menu items. At last, the fast American favorites have exposed their "fat facts."

Some fat facts

A McDonald's Big Mac has 530 calories, 28 grams of fat and 960 milligrams of sodium. Even the Filet-O-Fish has 360 calories, 16 grams of fat and 690 milligrams of sodium. Add French fries and a shake, and you're drowning in fat and sodium.

Three pieces of Kentucky Fried Chicken contain a whopping 790 calories, 51 grams of fat and 2285 milligrams of sodium. Add coleslaw, mashed potatoes with gravy and a biscuit, and you get a total of 1270 calories, 76 grams of fat and 3565 milligrams of sodium. That's over a full day's recommended allowance for both fat and sodium in just one meal, and 54% of the total calories come from fat!

Salads are usually considered a safe choice. However, many salads have close to 1000 calories, over 50 grams of fat, and over 1000 milligrams of sodium. Sometimes salads are higher in calories and fat than many other items on the menu.

Improvements in fast foods

In response to their new "fat visibility," most fast food restaurants quickly added items which look much better on the nutritional charts.

McDonald's makes a Fajita Chicken Salad and a Garden Salad, both under 170 calories and 7 grams of fat. Reduced calorie salad dressing is available. In addition, they have their McLean Deluxe sandwich, fat-free muffins, and low-fat frozen yogurt.

The Carl's Jr. Lite Menu offers a Charbroiled BBQ Chicken Sandwich with only 310 calories and 6 grams of fat. The Lite Menu also includes a Plain Potato, Garden Salad and Chicken Salad with reduced calorie salad dressing.

Jack In the Box serves a Chicken Fajita Pita with fewer than 300 calories and 8 grams of fat. Their Chicken Teriyaki Bowl contains lots of rice, which is very filling and very low in fat (1½ grams). They also serve low-fat milk and provide a reduced calorie salad dressing.

La Salsa specializes in fresh and healthy Mexican food, prepared without lard, and offers a unique salsa bar. Wendy's provides several low-fat choices, including their Garden Spot salad bar, grilled chicken sandwich, chili, and broccoli & cheese baked potatoes.

Consumer power

As a result of health-conscious consumers speaking out, we're now beginning to have the choice to "order healthy" at fast food restaurants. "The public does not realize the dramatic power it wields," Sokolof emphasizes. "The consumer's wish is big business' command."

But what about dining out in restaurants?

What's healthy and what's not?

If dining out were only for special occasions, the rich and creamy dishes could be wonderful treats. An occasional splurge might not be so bad. But as restaurant dining for business, pleasure and convenience becomes more common, it is important to find healthier choices.

That's what *Healthy Dining in Orange County* is all about. It's the first book of its kind. Never before has so much comprehensive information been available for restaurant menu items. Each restaurant has its own unique recipes, prepared in its own special way. So nutrition information must be compiled restaurant by restaurant, recipe by recipe. And that's a lot of work.

There are books which give general information for dining out. They list common entrees to avoid and those which are probably best to order. However, as restaurants become more specialized and creative, "common" entrees are not so common, so it's hard to follow those guidelines.

You can learn how to order healthy entrees by asking the right kinds of questions. *Healthy Dining* will make the process of ordering healthy food much easier, however.

As you read on about what we've discovered in our research, you'll find that often you can't tell what you're getting by the menu description. It may portray a healthy item, but many times there are hidden ingredients, and the method of preparation is not specified. Without complete nutrition information, you don't know what you're getting, and that can be dangerous!

Goals of *Healthy Dining in Orange County:*

1. To guide you in choosing low-fat, healthy entrees served at popular Orange County restaurants.

2. To provide you with easy-to-read nutrition profiles for the selected entrees.

3. To give you useful, practical guidelines and advice for healthier restaurant dining.

4. To encourage restaurants to prepare and serve a wide variety of healthy choices.

CHAPTER 2

Is Restaurant Food Fattening and Unhealthy?

It can be if you're not careful! But it doesn't have to be.

Many restaurants smother meals with excess fat, sodium, cholesterol and calories. Butter, oil, cream, cheese and salt are frequently added to achieve the taste and texture that the average American expects. To make matters worse, many restaurant diners have the habit of adding "extras" such as salad dressing, sour cream, and butter (which push up the calorie and fat count even more). Let's take a shocking look at a favorite restaurant dinner:

Chicken Breast
Topped with a Creamy Parmesan Sauce
Served with Dinner Salad, Baked Potato and Sauteed Vegetables

	Calories	Fat (g)	Cholest. (mg)	Sodium (mg)
Dinner Salad	32	0	0	53
Blue Cheese Dressing (4 Tbs)	308	32	36	668
Chicken Breast with Sauce	1312	91	481	1517
Baked Potato	220	0	0	16
Butter (2 Tbs)	200	23	61	232
Sour Cream (2 Tbs)	62	6	13	15
Sauteed Vegetables	117	11	0	207
Meal Total	2251	163	591	2708

Now let's evaluate these relative to daily recommendations:

Calories: Close to a FULL day's recommended calories <u>in one meal</u>.
Fat: <u>Almost three times</u> the recommended fat intake for a FULL Day.
Cholesterol: <u>Almost twice</u> the recommended cholesterol intake for a FULL Day.
Sodium: <u>Almost the entire</u> recommended sodium intake for a FULL Day.

Other fat-filled favorites:

	Calories	Fat (g)	Cholest. (mg)	Sodium (mg)
Italian manicotti with garlic bread	1393	79	411	2330
Beef & cheese enchiladas, rice & refried beans	1510	88	210	3516
Chicken fried steak with fries	1119	77	205	1895
Ultimate cheeseburger with fries & shake	1625	96	165	1708
Chicken sandwich with onion rings & shake	1282	68	82	2290
Seafood platter - fried - with tarter sauce	1195	70	97	1780
Salmon - smothered in a cream sauce	1024	76	283	1017
Fried chicken - with potato salad & cole slaw	1124	71	239	2552
Stir fry chicken with rice & egg rolls	1213	62	99	2907
Lasagna with garlic bread & salad	1538	77	194	2805
Omelet with hashbrowns	850	53	892	852
Pizza - sausage & mushroom	1290	48	84	1656
Chimichanga with sour cream & cheese	922	68	205	2125
Salad bar - with potato & tuna salad, dressing, and muffins with butter	1715	89	310	2954

Does dining out have to be so destructive to our health?

Some say, "Order grilled fish, salads or vegetarian dishes. By avoiding red meat, fried foods and creamy sauces, you can dine out and stay on your diet."

Be careful! We've analyzed hundreds of apparently "healthy" entrees and found that many were diet disasters. Frequently, "healthy" dishes are laced with unhealthy, hidden ingredients. The menu descriptions portray a healthy item, but when we looked into the preparation methods, we found the items contained too much of certain unhealthy ingredients.

Surprising nutrition information about apparently "healthy" meals:

Grilled Swordfish - *Marinated in herbs and olive oil.*

884	Calories	
71	Fat (g)	Over a full day's recommended fat intake.
115	Cholesterol (mg)	Too much olive oil used in the preparation!
846	Sodium (mg)	

Vegetarian Pasta Primavera - *Fresh vegetables and garlic sauteed in a vegetable broth. Served over fettucini noodles and tossed with Parmesan cheese.*

816	Calories	The menu description didn't mention that the
45	Fat (g)	pasta was heavily tossed with oil, and the
139	Cholesterol (mg)	vegetables were sauteed in both broth *and*
892	Sodium (mg)	*butter.* This brings the fat total to 75% of
		a FULL day's recommended fat intake.

The "Healthy" Sandwich - *Avocado, tomato & cheese on whole wheat bread.*

746	Calories	
50	Fat (g)	This is a healthy sandwich?
66	Cholesterol (mg)	Avocado, cheese, and mayonnaise add
958	Sodium (mg)	up to too much fat and sodium.

Cobb Salad - *Crispy greens topped with chicken, avocado, bacon, tomato, hard-boiled egg and blue cheese crumbles. Served with a generous portion of your favorite dressing.*

1296	Calories	
102	Fat (g)	Very unhealthy. Much too high in fat,
647	Cholesterol (mg)	cholesterol, sodium and calories.
2553	Sodium (mg)	

Shrimp Stirfry - *Shrimp and assorted vegetables with chow mein noodles.*

866	Calories	Too much fat, calories, cholesterol and sodium.
64	Fat (g)	1 oz. oil to saute (27 g fat), butter/cream
392	Cholesterol (mg)	sauce (25 g fat), and the chow mein noodles
668	Sodium (mg)	(9 g fat) quickly add up.

Tostada - *Mexican beans, guacamole, lettuce, tomato and cheese.*

1416	Calories	
77	Fat (g)	The cheese alone contributes 519 calories,
288	Cholesterol (mg)	43 grams of fat, 137 mg cholesterol and
2010	Sodium (mg)	802 mg sodium.

We also found other items labeled "Light" or "Light-Fare" that included potato skins (deep fried), vegetables with cheese sauce, a hamburger patty and cottage cheese (too much saturated fat), cheese quesadillas (there's that saturated fat in the cheese again) and deep fried fish tacos.

Remember: It's all in the preparation

You can't tell enough about menu items by just reading the menu description. The preparation method also determines how healthy an entree is. If you're concerned about what goes into your body, you must rely on complete nutrition information, not just a menu description.

WARNING:

The ♥ used on menus does not necessarily mean the item is low in calories, fat or sodium.

What you don't know _CAN_ hurt you!

If you rely on the ♥ listed on restaurant menus to guide you in choosing healthy entrees, you may be gambling with your health. Don't automatically assume that these entrees are approved by the American Heart Association or other health organizations, because usually they are not. The symbol is simply an indication that the restaurant considers it a healthy choice.

Unfortunately, in almost all cases, these items have never been nutritionally analyzed. In fact, when Accents On Health analyzed entrees with a ♥ next to them, we discovered that many were too high in fat. Here are a few examples:

??? Heart Healthy Entrees ???

♥	Eggplant Salad	34 grams fat - 86% of calories from fat
♥	Pasta with Tomatoes & Garlic	42 grams fat - 50% of calories from fat
♥	Greens Topped with Grilled Ahi	26 grams fat - 73% of calories from fat
♥	Grilled Halibut	64 grams fat - 75% of calories from fat

Is all restaurant food fattening & unhealthy?

_NO!_ Many restaurants in Orange County are preparing delightfully delicious entrees which are wonderfully good for you! Instead of smothering foods with excessive amounts of unhealthy ingredients, they've creatively used herbs, spices, small amounts of unsaturated oils and healthy preparation methods. They have your health _and_ your tastebuds in mind.

Some scrumptious and healthy examples:

Garden Bistro (Costa Mesa)
SAUTEED BARBERRIES & CURRANTS IN SAFFRON RICE & MARINATED BREAST OF CHICKEN

✓ CALORIES: Low (599)　　　　✓ CHOLESTEROL: Low (87 mg)
✓✓ FAT: Very Low (9 g)　　　　✓✓ SODIUM: Very Low (83 mg) **

Walt's Wharf (Seal Beach)
ORANGE ROUGHY WITH PAPAYA AND RED CHILE SALSA
with steamed vegetables and baked potato (request plain).

✓ CALORIES: Low (394)　　　　✓✓ CHOLESTEROL: Very Low (45 mg)
✓✓ FAT: Very Low* (4 g)　　　　✓✓ SODIUM: Very Low (163 mg) **

Il Fornaio (Irvine)
FUSILLI AI VEGETALI
Corkscrew pasta, fresh vegetables and herbs (no butter or oil).

✓ CALORIES: Low (540)　　　　✓✓ CHOLESTEROL: Very Low (4 mg)
✓ FAT: Low* (3 g)　　　　✓✓ SODIUM: Very Low (319 mg) **

Ferdussi Taste of Persia (Santa Ana)
WHITE FISH KABOB
Fresh filet of white fish dipped in saffron sauce and cooked on open flame.

✓✓ CALORIES: Very Low (317)　　　　✓ CHOLESTEROL: Low (112 mg)
✓✓ FAT: Very Low* (6 g)　　　　✓✓ SODIUM: Very Low (257 mg) **

Daily's (Laguna Hills, Laguna Niguel & Tustin)
BOWL OF 3-BEAN & CORN CHILI (VEGETARIAN)
Served on brown rice with a dollop of yogurt and green salad.

✓✓ CALORIES: Very Low (283)　　✓✓ CHOLESTEROL: None (0 mg)
✓✓ FAT: Very Low* (3½ g)　　　　✓ SODIUM: Low (350 mg)

Five Crowns (Corona del Mar)
PORCINI MUSHROOM RAVIOLI
Tossed with fresh tomatoes, basil, garlic and extra virgin olive oil.

✓ CALORIES: Low (372)　　　　✓✓ CHOLESTEROL: Very Low (50 mg)
✓ FAT: Low (14 g)　　　　✓ SODIUM: Low (456 mg) **

* Primarily unsaturated fat
** If you request no added salt

Some scrumptious and healthy examples (continued):

Veg à Go-Go (Newport Beach)
THAI RAP

Spicy Thai vinaigrette, fresh cilantro, bean sprouts, carrots, broccoli & red cabbage in a low-fat tortilla.

✓✓ CALORIES: Very Low (248) ✓✓ CHOLESTEROL: None (0 mg)
✓✓ FAT: Very Low* (9 g) ✓ SODIUM: Low (407 mg)

Round Table Pizza (25 Orange County locations)
SALUTÉ CASHEW CHICKEN PIZZA (2 SLICES)

Sweet & spicy Oriental chili sauce, 3 cheeses, roasted chicken, roasted cashews, pineapple, zucchini, green peppers, carrots, yellow onions, garlic, Roma tomatoes & green onions. Analysis for 2 slices large pizza.

✓✓ CALORIES: Very Low (300) ✓✓ CHOLESTEROL: Very Low (30 mg)
✓✓ FAT: Very Low (8 g) ✓ SODIUM: Low (480 mg)

Palm Court at the Waterfront Hilton Beach Resort (Huntington Beach)
HERB SEARED TUNA TRIANGLES

Served chilled around rice noodles with a Thai curry sauce.

✓✓ CALORIES: Very Low (282) ✓ CHOLESTEROL: Low (97 mg)
✓✓ FAT: Very Low (8 g) ✓✓ SODIUM: Very Low (274 mg) **

The menu items above and in the following chapters are just a taste of the wonderful entrees served at the restaurants participating in **Healthy Dining in Orange County.** We invite you to visit the restaurants featured in this book. You'll discover a whole new world of menu items that are marvelously delicious and so good for you!

---

* Primarily unsaturated fat
** If you request no added salt

"Special Requests"

In some cases, after we analyzed the restaurant recipes, we found dishes that contained too many calories and/or too much fat, cholesterol or sodium. So we recommended that the chef modify the dishes to meet the *Healthy Dining* guidelines. We note these dishes as "Special Requests." "Special Requests" may be prepared with less oil or butter, salad dressing or sauce served on the side, less cheese, etc. When you order, you must ask for the "Special Request" to make it correspond to the published nutrition information. See the examples below to find out how many calories and grams of fat you save by ordering some of these "Special Requests."

Examples of "Special Requests:"

Milano's (Irvine)
TAGLIATELLE DEL GIARDINO - SPECIAL REQUEST
Fettuccine with julienned seasonal vegetables tossed in a white wine and tomato-basil sauce. Request no butter or oil. This "Special Request" saves 441 calories, 50 grams of fat, 62 mg cholesterol and 235 mg sodium.

Ruby's Diner (14 Orange County locations)
CHICKEN RUBYBURGER - SPECIAL REQUEST
with a tender, boneless, skinless chicken breast. Request no margarine or mayonnaise. This "Special Request" saves 300 calories, 33 grams of fat, 12 mg cholesterol and 316 mg sodium.

Palm Court at the Waterfront Hilton Beach Resort (Huntington Beach)
ANGELO DI CIELO - SPECIAL REQUEST
Angel hair pasta, shrimp, crab claws, peas, fresh herbs, tomato, olive oil and parmesan. Request less oil (½ oz). This "Special Request" saves 875 calories and 99 grams of fat.

Mark's (Laguna Beach)
MEDALLIONS OF TURKEY - SPECIAL REQUEST
Sautéed, with lemon, butter and capers, and served with vegetables. Request no butter and vegetables steamed. This "Special Request" saves over 200 calories and 23 grams of fat.

Rutabegorz (Fullerton, Irvine & Tustin)
VEGGIE SURPRISE - SPECIAL REQUEST
A combo of fresh veggies & sunflower seeds on top a mound of rice pilaf. Request no cheese. This "Special Request" saves 505 calories, 40 grams of fat, 121 mg cholesterol and 919 mg sodium.

Examples of "Special Requests" (continued):

Michael's Supper Club (Dana Point)
GREEK SALAD - SPECIAL REQUEST
Fresh crisp greens tossed with roma tomatoes, chopped bell peppers, Bermuda onions, cucumbers, calamata olives, Feta cheese and our Grecian herb dressing. Request dressing on the side (not included in analysis). This "Special Request" saves 527 calories and 57 grams of fat.

California Pizza Kitchen (Irvine, Laguna Hills, Mission Viejo, Santa Ana & Newport Beach)
BROCCOLI SUNDRIED TOMATO FUSILLI - SPECIAL REQUEST
Corkscrew pasta with fresh broccoli, browned garlic, sun-dried tomatoes, fresh thyme and Parmesan cheese. Request no oil. This "Special Request" saves 357 calories and 41 grams of fat.

Mon Chateau (Lake Forest)
POULET AUX FINES HERBES - SPECIAL REQUEST
A supreme, gratifying breast of chicken with fine herbs intensified by a white wine chicken velouté. Request less oil (¼ oz) and no butter. This "Special Request" saves 280 calories and 32 grams of fat.

Remember: Any dish marked "Special Request" means you must specifically order the "Special Request" to make it correspond to the published nutrition information.

CHAPTER 3

Do Your Calories Have a Purpose?

Calories have a bad reputation in our society. We're counting calories and cutting calories, as though we've forgotten that calories are what keep us alive. Food and water fuel our bodies to do the miraculous tasks we perform each day. Instead of focusing on just cutting calories, we need to look at the *quality* of the calories we consume.

Just what are you getting from your calories?

Calories add up from the amounts of protein, carbohydrate and fat in foods. Each type of calorie has a very different function in the body. The following chapters explain the functions in more detail, but briefly:

Protein calories help the body to build and restore.

Carbohydrate calories are the body's main energy source.

Fat calories turn to fat -- *easily*.

In general, protein and carbohydrate calories supply our bodies with nutrients necessary to function optimally. We need a very small amount of fat each day, but because fat is very easy to get, most Americans suffer from an excess of dietary fat, not a deficiency.

We should strive to eat foods with high-quality, nutritious calories. Recommendations vary according to individual needs, but generally 50% to 65% of total daily calories should come from carbohydrates, 10% to 20% from protein, and 15% to 30% from fat. Because most Americans get enough protein and too much fat, the best way to determine the quality of your calories is to determine the percentage of calories from fat, and keep it under 30%.

Percentage of calories from fat

It's important to note that the 30% fat recommendation is the suggested average for the whole day. Over the day, some foods will add little, if any, fat to your diet, while other foods may supply a big chunk of the fat for the day. Of course, it's best to avoid (or use sparingly) foods which have a high percentage of fat (e.g. butter, margarine, oils, sour cream, cheese, cream cheese, etc.).

A fattening example:

Salmon - *Smothered in a cream sauce*
    Total Calories: 1024
    Protein   77 grams
    Carbohydrate   8 grams
    Fat   76 grams

How to calculate the percentage of calories from fat:

Each gram of fat has nine calories. Using this information, you can calculate the percent of calories from fat as shown in the following example. For the **Salmon with Cream Sauce** listed above:

1. Multiply the number of grams of fat by 9 (number of calories per gram of fat):
    76 grams x 9 cals/gram = 684 calories from fat

2. Divide by total calories and multiply by 100 to get the percentage:
    684 calories ÷ 1024 calories x 100 = 67%

67% of calories in this dish come from fat!

Carbohydrate and protein percentages can be calculated in a similar way, except that the number of grams of each is multiplied by 4 rather than 9, because carbohydrates and proteins have 4 calories per gram. The division step is the same. For this example, these calculations show that 3% of calories come from carbohydrate and 30% from protein. Cholesterol and sodium do not contribute to calories.

The small percentage of carbohydrate is common for meat, poultry, and fish entrees, but a nutritious entree should contain less fat. In this example, most of the fat comes from the cream and butter used in the sauce; however, it's not necessary to add excess fat to get a delicious tasting entree.

Let's look at a healthier salmon dish:

Salmon Teriyaki (Amachi Japanese Restaurant - Costa Mesa)

    Total Calories: 343
    Protein   39 grams
    Carbohydrates   14 grams
    Fat   12 grams

To calculate the percentage of calories from fat:

1. Multiply grams of fat by 9 calories per gram:
   12 grams x 9 cals/gram = 108 calories from fat

2. Divide by total calories and multiply by 100 to get a percentage:
   108 calories ÷ 343 calories x 100 = 31

31% of calories in this dish come from fat, slightly above the recommended limit.

Remember, the guideline of 30% or fewer calories from fat applies to the entire day, not just one entree. Also, restaurants differ greatly in what they include as side dishes with meals. If you order a lean meat or fish entree, it consists mainly of protein and fat, and the percentage of fat will generally appear to be high. By themselves, many lean meats and fish contain 30% to 40% fat. Even soybeans contain about 40% of their calories from fat. But generally these high-protein entrees are not eaten by themselves. If you choose quality carbohydrate side dishes such as vegetables, grains, breads, and fruits, the percentage of fat for the overall meal will be significantly less. Entrees which are made up largely of carbohydrates (such as pasta or rice dishes) will generally have a lower percentage of calories from fat, unless loaded with excess oil, butter, cream, etc.

As an example of how a side dish can change the overall percentage fat, let's include the rice that is served with this meal:

	Calories	Fat (g)
Salmon Teriyaki	343	12
Rice (1 cup)	205	0
Total	548	12

To calculate percentage of calories from fat:

12 grams of fat x 9 cals/gram = 108 calories from fat
108 calories from fat ÷ 548 total calories x 100 = 20%

Only 20% of total calories in this meal come from fat, which is well within the recommended guidelines and significantly less than the percentage of fat calculated for only the entree by itself.

This example of the salmon demonstrates how a healthy entree, although near or slightly above the recommended 30% fat limit, can still be an excellent choice. It's protein-rich, and it also contains "good," unsaturated fat. Remember that a meal like this will probably be the largest of your day, and your choices for the remainder of the day can also bring down the overall percentage of calories from fat.

Grams of fat vs. percentage of calories from fat

We list grams of fat for each of the dishes on the menu pages rather than percentage of calories from fat. The example above illustrates how calculating the percentage of calories from fat for only a single menu item does not adequately reflect values for the entire meal or the entire day. Instead, if you total the grams of fat for each meal, you can more accurately determine your daily fat intake. Chapter 4 discusses in more detail how to choose guidelines for fat intake that are appropriate for you.

How the check mark guidelines for calories were set:

We set the guidelines assuming an average intake of 2,000 calories per day. Next, we assumed that the restaurant meal accounts for the largest of the day's meals, or at least 1/3 of the daily total calories. So 600 calories for the main entree would fit into the calorie budget. Thus, 600 calories is labeled as "Low" in calories. The "Very Low" value of 350 calories represents a proportionally lower level, corresponding to about 1200 calories per day:

✓✓ Very Low = 0 to 350 calories/entree
✓ Low = 350 to 600 calories/entree

> Glance through the restaurant pages and use the quick, easy check mark system to see the wide variety of entrees which contain high-quality, nutritious calories and are low (✓) or very low (✓✓) in total calories.

CHAPTER 4

Fat - How Much and What Type?

Fat -- clogging our arteries and building up around the stomach, thighs and buttocks. Too much body fat, almost always caused by too much fat in our diet and too little exercise in our day, increases the risks of high blood pressure, elevated blood fats (triglycerides and cholesterol), heart disease, stroke, diabetes, cancer and other health problems.

How much is too much?

The guidelines recommended by the American Heart Association and the Surgeon General's Office (see Chapter 1) suggest that fat should contribute no more than 30% of total calories. Chapter 3 shows examples of calculating percentage of calories from fat. This section deals with counting grams of fat. If we assume a daily intake of 2000 calories, then no more than 600 calories per day (30%) should come from fat. Since each gram of fat contributes nine calories, then about 66 grams of fat (600 ÷ 9) is the suggested upper limit of fat intake per day. If you're not careful, it's very easy to exceed that with just one meal!

What is a reasonable limit per meal or per entree? If we divide the day's allotment (66 grams) into three equal meals, then a reasonable limit per meal is 22 grams of fat. Main entrees usually contribute the largest amount of fat to the meal (unless you load your side dishes with too much fat, as discussed below), so we set guidelines of:

✓✓ "Very Low" = 0 to 10 grams of fat/entree
✓ "Low" = 10 to 20 grams of fat/entree

If you're very active and take in more calories, then a higher limit would be appropriate. If you're on a weight loss diet or very low fat diet, then the "Very Low" guideline of up to 10 grams of fat per entree is probably more appropriate.

Notice that these recommended guidelines represent an average intake for an average meal. Don't be overly concerned about the cutoff between our designations of "Low" and "Very Low." Unless you're on a very restricted diet, the difference between an entree with 11 grams of fat (which would receive one check mark) and one with 9 grams of fat (two check marks) is probably not worth worrying about. An occasional meal with somewhat more fat (but don't overdo it!) can be fairly easily compensated for by reducing fat intake during other meals.

Be aware of portion sizes. Some people remember food labels on products which list only 2 or 3 grams of fat, and so they consider 9 or 10 grams of fat unthinkable! However, those 2 or 3 grams of fat may correspond to only a one-ounce serving size. The entrees listed in this book often represent 6 - 10 ounces of a <u>very filling</u>, protein-rich meal. Even 20 grams of fat is <u>much</u> lower than most typical restaurant meals (see Chapter 2) and will probably still fit within your daily limit. You may also choose to eat a smaller serving and save some for later.

Types of fat:

Together with protein, fats form the structures in our bodies, including muscles, nerves, membranes and blood vessels. We need very little fat to perform these functions, and only *unsaturated* sources of fat aid in these processes. "Saturated" and "unsaturated" refer to the chemical structure of the fat molecules.

<u>Saturated Fats</u>.   Saturated fats are the <u>*very unhealthy*</u> fats which raise blood cholesterol levels. Excess saturated fat is related to an increased risk of cardiovascular disease. Foods that contain saturated fats are usually hard at room temperature. Saturated fat is found mostly in animal products (beef, chicken, butter, ice cream, cheese), processed and fast foods and some vegetable oils (palm oil, coconut oil, partially hydrogenated oils).

<u>Unsaturated Fats - Monounsaturated, Polyunsaturated</u>. These are the *"good"* types of fat. A <u>low total fat intake</u>, with the majority of fat from unsaturated sources, appears to lower blood cholesterol levels. The best sources for these "good" fats are natural grains, seeds and nuts, and fish. Many oils are primarily unsaturated, such as olive, canola, peanut, corn, safflower, sesame, cottonseed and soybean. Once again, these fats are "good" only in very small amounts! Look for menu items with the * for dishes that contain primarily unsaturated fat.

<u>Hydrogenated Fats</u>. The vegetable oils found in many packaged or processed foods are hydrogenated. The process of hydrogenation changes the chemical structure of unsaturated fats by adding hydrogen atoms to make the fats more saturated. Manufacturers use the hydrogenation process because it increases product stability and shelf life. Thus, a larger quantity can be produced at one time, saving the manufacturer money. Unfortunately, this money-saving process contributes to elevated blood cholesterol levels and increases heart disease risk.

<u>Omega-3 Fats</u>. Some types of fish contain unique polyunsaturated fats called Omega-3 fatty acids. These fatty acids seem to make blood platelets less likely to clot, thus decreasing risk of artery blockage and heart attack. Fish with high amounts of Omega-3 include salmon, albacore tuna, mackerel, herring and rainbow trout.

A summary of fat:

When assessing the fat content of food, it is important to look at:
1. The number of grams of fat
2. The percentage of calories from fat
3. The type of fat - minimize or avoid saturated fats

One Last Word on Fat: Unsaturated fats do not raise blood cholesterol levels. But too much fat -- saturated or unsaturated -- may make you fat, and excess body fat is a risk factor for many chronic diseases.

> On the restaurant menu pages, the asterisk (*) next to the grams of fat indicates that the fat is primarily unsaturated (the "good" type). Look for it!

Some delicious "Very Low" fat examples:

Notice that many contain primarily unsaturated fat (designated with the *).

Spaghettini (Seal Beach)
CIOPPINO DEL MARE
A larger terrine of our cioppino style soup brimming with shrimp, grilled fresh fish and fresh seasonal shellfish over risotto.
✓✓ FAT: Very Low* (8 g)

Elephant Bar (Laguna Hills)
SIZZLING CHICKEN FAJITAS
Marinated skinless chicken breast charbroiled over peppers and onions. Served with ranch beans, salsa, shredded lettuce & warm corn tortillas.
✓✓ FAT: Very Low (8 g)

John Dominis (Newport Beach)
TIGER PRAWNS STIR-FRIED IN BLACK BEAN SAUCE
Large succulent prawns stir-fried in black beans, and served with steamed vegetables and rice (rice not included in analysis).
✓✓ FAT: Very Low* (10 g)

Brazilian Tropical Cafe (Newport Beach)
SPICY BAHIA CREPE (REGULAR SIZE)
Sautéed shrimp in spicy Bahia sauce (tomato & mushroom) with rice.
✓✓ FAT: Very Low* (4 g)

Now - how well are YOU doing?

Now that Orange County restaurants are watching how much fat they're adding to your diet, just _how well are you watching?_ Here are some easy ways to add too much fat to your diet - quickly!

High-fat culprits:

	Calories	Fat (g)	Cholest. (mg)	Sodium (mg)
Salad Dressings: (3 Tbs.)				
Blue Cheese	231	24	27	501
Thousand Island	176	17	15	327
French	201	19	6	642
Italian	206	21	0	348
Oil & Vinegar	215	24	0	0
Toppings: (2 Tbs)				
Butter	200	23	61	232
Margarine	202	23	0	264
Sour Cream	67	6	13	15
Cream Cheese	100	10	31	85
Tarter Sauce	150	16	18	196
Mayonnaise	198	22	16	157
Cheese (1 oz. cheddar)	114	9	30	176
Desserts:				
Cheesecake	386	24	82	284
Apple Pie	323	14	28	207
Chocolate Cake	407	17	5	300
Ice Cream (1 cup)	349	24	88	108

Instead try:

- Fat-free or low-fat salad dressings
- Salsa, low-fat cottage cheese, or yogurt as salad dressing or topping for potatoes
- Only very small amounts of regular or high-fat salad dressings
- Frozen yogurt, sorbet, sherbet or fruit for dessert

CHAPTER 5

Cholesterol - A Hot Topic

Cholesterol continues to be a hot topic enmeshed in controversy. Medical research is progressing on this subject, and we hope to clear up some misconceptions concerning cholesterol.

Where does cholesterol come from?

Most of the cholesterol in your blood is manufactured by your liver. The body produces about 1,000 milligrams (mg.) of cholesterol each day. In addition, the average American consumes 400 to 600 mg. from food (animal products) each day. The cholesterol we derive from our diets is essentially the same as the cholesterol our bodies manufacture. Our bodies use cholesterol to form hormones and cell membranes.

However, the average high-fat/high-cholesterol diet tends to add too much cholesterol to the bloodstream. The excess cholesterol and other substances accumulate in the walls of the blood vessels. Over time the arteries become narrowed, and eventually the flow of blood is cut off, leading to a heart attack or stroke.

How should blood cholesterol be measured?

To get an accurate and complete cholesterol measure, a tube of blood should be drawn from the arm by a qualified health professional. You should not eat or drink anything (except water) for 12 hours before the blood draw. The laboratory which analyzes the blood sample should follow the reference methods set by the U. S. Centers For Disease Control. The fingertip method found in shopping malls and health fairs may not provide results that are as accurate.

What determines blood cholesterol levels?

1. **Genetics**. Some individuals, no matter how prudent their diet or how regularly they exercise, can't achieve a low cholesterol level without the help of a physician and cholesterol-lowering medications.

2. **Lipoproteins**. Cholesterol is carried through the blood in protein packages called lipoproteins. The amounts and types of lipoproteins are an important indicator of your heart disease risk.

LDLs (low-density lipoproteins) are commonly termed "bad" cholesterol. LDLs increase heart disease risk because they keep cholesterol in blood circulation and carry it to the arteries to be deposited. Excess body fat and a diet high in saturated fat tend to increase LDL levels.

HDLs (high-density lipoproteins) are the "good" cholesterol that protect against heart disease. They actually carry cholesterol AWAY from the arteries to the liver to be excreted from the body. Individuals with high HDL levels have a lower risk of heart disease. Regular exercise, maintaining appropriate body weight, and not smoking help to increase HDL levels.

3. **Diet**. Foods high in saturated fat _increase_ cholesterol levels. These include: butter, whole milk products, palm and coconut oils, cheese, beef, pork, and eggs. In addition, many packaged and processed foods are high in saturated fat or (partially) hydrogenated oils, which also have a cholesterol-raising effect.

A diet _low in total fat_, with fat intake primarily from unsaturated fat sources, _reduces_ cholesterol levels. Unsaturated fats include: olive, corn, safflower, sesame, canola, soybean, and sunflower oils. _High fiber foods_, especially oat bran, apples, carrots, oranges, legumes (beans, peas and lentils) _decrease_ cholesterol levels by inhibiting the absorption of cholesterol into the bloodstream. _Fish and fish oils_, which contain omega-3 fatty acids, also _decrease_ cholesterol levels.

4. **Smoking, stress and some medications** also raise cholesterol levels.

Important facts on dietary cholesterol and fat:

Too much of any fat (even unsaturated oils!) can increase body fat, and excess body fat may increase blood cholesterol levels. Oils, margarine, and butter all have approximately the same number of calories and fat grams per ounce, and so all have the same potential to make you fat. Therefore it's important to limit your total intake of all types of fat.

Even though oils, margarine, and butter have about the same calorie and fat counts, there is a big difference in the chemical make-up of these fats. Butter contains saturated fat, and saturated fats increase blood cholesterol levels. Saturated fats stimulate the production of LDLs ("bad cholesterol"), resulting in increased blood cholesterol levels. Therefore if you avoid only dietary cholesterol in the food you eat, without reducing the amount of saturated fat, you may not decrease your blood cholesterol level at all.

Avoid hydrogenated fats too, because they are also saturated. Margarine, although cholesterol-free, is partially hydrogenated and contains trans-fatty acids, which have been shown to have a cholesterol-raising effect.

Vegetable oils are generally <u>unsaturated fats</u>. Liquid oils (such as olive, corn, canola, etc.) in small amounts may help to decrease cholesterol levels. Remember though, that all oils are 100% fat, so use only small amounts.

The <u>amount of cholesterol</u> found in foods is not as important as the <u>amount of saturated fat</u>. But you should minimize intake of very concentrated sources of cholesterol such as egg yolks and liver. Shellfish is very low in saturated fat, but moderately high in cholesterol. Most medical experts agree that shellfish, in small quantities, is a healthy choice.

Cholesterol is found only in animal products. Don't be misled, though. Products which don't contain cholesterol may still be loaded with fat. Food packages stating "No Cholesterol" should alert you to look at the nutrition information on the label to determine the amount of total and saturated fat.

How the check mark guidelines for cholesterol were chosen:

The Surgeon General's Office and the American Heart Association recommend that cholesterol consumption be limited to 300 mg. per day. If the day's total were evenly divided in thirds, this would suggest a limit of 100 mg. per meal. We set our guidelines for cholesterol as follows:

> ✓✓ Very Low = 0 to 75 mg cholesterol/entree
> ✓ Low = 75 to 150 mg cholesterol/entree

If every meal in your day were at the "Low" limit of 150 mg, you would exceed the recommended amount. But since a restaurant meal usually contains a larger portion of meat or other cholesterol-containing foods than side dishes or other meals of the day, we assumed that this cholesterol intake can easily be compensated for by choosing foods with little or no cholesterol for the remaining selections.

If you are watching your blood cholesterol level, select items which are:

1. "Very Low" fat or "Low" fat
2. Primarily unsaturated (designated with the *)
3. "Very Low" or "Low" cholesterol

Some flavorful "Very Low" and "Low" cholesterol examples:

Tutto Mare (Newport Beach)
VERMICELLI AGLI SCAMPI
Thin spaghetti, langostino, baby clams, brandy & tomato sauce.
✓✓ FAT: Very Low* (10 g)   ✓ CHOLESTEROL: Low (95 mg)

Flavorful "Very Low" and "Low" cholesterol examples (continued):

T.G.I. Friday's (Brea, Costa Mesa, Laguna Niguel & Orange)
PACIFIC COAST TUNA
A medley of steamed fresh seasonal vegetables with slices of charbroiled tuna steak atop linguini. Served with fat-free plum sauce or oriental vinaigrette for dipping.
✓✓ FAT: Very Low (7½ g)   ✓✓ CHOLESTEROL: Very Low (70 mg)

Frankly Grill (Laguna Niguel)
VEGETARIAN HOT DOG
✓✓ FAT: Very Low* (4 g)   ✓✓ CHOLESTEROL: None (0 mg)

Gringa's Grill (Balboa Island)
CHICKEN SOFT TACO
A flour tortilla filled with chopped cabbage, cotija cheese, green onions and chicken.
✓✓ FAT: Very Low (7 g)   ✓✓ CHOLESTEROL: Very Low (37 mg)

Mother's Market & Kitchen (Costa Mesa, Huntington Beach & Irvine)
MA'S CHILI
Ma's homemade high protein remedy in an authentic zesty sauce. (14 oz bowl).
✓✓ FAT: Very Low* (2 g)   ✓✓ CHOLESTEROL: None (0 mg)

Charley Brown's (Anaheim)
FRESH SNAPPER WITH "SIMPLY LIGHT" TOPPING
Covered in a light tomato-basil vinaigrette.
✓ FAT: Low* (14 g)   ✓ CHOLESTEROL: Low (82 mg)

Nieuport 17 (Tustin)
SPAGHETTI WITH FRESH TOMATO COULIS
✓✓ FAT: Very Low* (9 g)   ✓✓ CHOLESTEROL: None (0 mg)

Sizzler (27 Orange County locations)
LEMON-HERB CHICKEN OR HIBACHI CHICKEN
Tender 8 oz chicken breast seasoned in lemon and herbs or basted with Hibachi sauce.
✓✓ FAT: Very Low (5 g)   ✓ CHOLESTEROL: Low (134 mg)

Marrakesh (Newport Beach)
VEGETABLE COUSCOUS
Steamed cracked wheat topped with fresh vegetables and raisins.
✓✓ FAT: Very Low* (6 g)   ✓✓ CHOLESTEROL: None (0 mg)

* Primarily unsaturated fat

CHAPTER 6

Sodium - To Salt or Not to Salt?

That is the question. Sodium is an essential nutrient. It helps to maintain blood volume, regulate the balance of water in the cells, and transmit nerve impulses. The kidneys control sodium balance by increasing or decreasing sodium in the urine.

In general, Americans consume more sodium than the body needs. Many foods contain sodium naturally, and it is commonly added to foods during preparation or processing. Sodium is also found in drinking water, prescription drugs and over-the-counter medications.

One teaspoon of salt contains about 2,000 milligrams of sodium, approximately 2/3 of the American Heart Association's recommended daily amount. Other condiments contain significant amounts of sodium, such as seasoning salts (1620 - 1850 mg. per teaspoon), monosodium glutamate -- MSG (492 mg. per teaspoon), soy sauce (343 mg. per teaspoon), and meat tenderizer (1750 mg. per teaspoon). Packaged and processed foods also tend to be very high in sodium.

In the United States, about one in four adults has elevated blood pressure. Sodium intake is only one of the factors known to affect high blood pressure, and not everyone is equally susceptible. The sensitivity to sodium seems to be very individualized. At present, there is not a good method to predict who is salt-sensitive or who will develop high blood pressure. Low-sodium diets may help some people avoid high blood pressure. Low-sodium diets may help some people with high blood pressure to control their blood pressure. And in some individuals, a low-sodium diet will not affect blood pressure at all.

Since most Americans consume more sodium than needed, consider reducing your sodium intake. Use less table salt, read labels carefully, and eat sparingly those foods which have large amounts of sodium. Remember that a substantial amount of the sodium you eat may be "hidden" -- either occurring naturally in foods or as part of a preservative or flavoring agent that has been added.

To avoid too much sodium:

- Learn to enjoy the flavors of unsalted foods.
- Cook without salt or with only small amounts of added salt.
- Flavor foods with herbs, spices, and lemon juice.
- Add little or no salt to food at the table.
- Limit your intake of salty foods such as potato chips, pretzels, salted nuts and popcorn, condiments (soy sauce, steak sauce, garlic salt), pickled foods, cured meats, cheeses, and canned foods.
- Read food labels carefully to determine the amounts of sodium.
- Use lower sodium products, when available, to replace those with higher sodium content.

To avoid too much sodium when dining out:

1. Order entrees with "Low" or "Very Low" sodium levels, and
2. Request no added salt whenever possible.

The analyses shown in this book reflect the sodium content that occurs naturally in food, as well as salt that is included in a prepared sauce or recipe where the sodium cannot be reduced for an individual portion. In addition, many chefs cook with salt "to taste" that is not included in the recipes they provided for analysis. Therefore it's important to specify very clearly that you want "no added salt."

> The double asterisk (**) next to the sodium values reminds you to specify "no added salt" to get the values as published.

Note: Many items included in this book are listed as "moderate" (meaning 600 to 1000 mg sodium per entree) or "high" in sodium (meaning above 1000 mg sodium per entree) and are not recommended for those watching sodium intake.

How the check mark guidelines for sodium were set:

Of the 3000 mg. of sodium recommended per day, we consider a value of 1000 mg. per meal (1/3 of 3000) to be a reasonable level. We assume 600 mg can reasonably come from the main entree as a "Low" value, and the remainder from side dishes. A "Very Low" level is ½ of the "Low" value, or 300 mg:

✓✓ Very Low = 0 to 300 mg sodium/entree
✓ Low = 350 to 600 mg sodium/entree

Some splendid "Very Low" and "Low" sodium examples:

Antonello (Santa Ana)
FUSILI AI FILETTI DI POMODORO
Corkscrew pasta with fresh tomato fillets, garlic and basil sauce.
✓✓ SODIUM: Very Low (46 mg) **

Chimayo (Newport Beach)
BBQ SALMON IN CORN HUSK
Salmon topped with Poblano pesto and corn salsa, and served with vegetable medley.
✓ SODIUM: Low (387 mg) **

Bukhara Cuisine of India (Huntington Beach)
KARAHI CHICKEN (½ SERVING)
Chicken cooked in juice of garlic, ginger and tomatoes.
✓✓ SODIUM: Very Low (88 mg) **

Villa Roma (Lake Forest)
CAPELLINI ALLA CHECCA
Angel hair pasta with fresh chopped tomato, garlic and fresh basil.
✓✓ SODIUM: Very Low (92 mg) **

Gustav's Jägerhaus (Anaheim)
"ROCK" FISH (COD)
Cook it yourself on a greaseless tabletop stone.
✓✓ SODIUM: Very Low (137 mg) **

** If you request no added salt

CHAPTER 7

Protein, Carbs, & Diabetic Exchanges

Protein: the building blocks

Protein is very important for a healthy body. Protein provides materials for growth, helps to maintain and repair tissues, manufactures the lipoproteins to carry fat, and assists in the maintenance of proper fluid levels.

It is very easy to get protein in our diet, and most Americans consume 2 - 3 times more than necessary. Excess protein does not create muscle, as many hope, but is stored as fat. Excess protein puts a strain on the liver and kidneys. In addition, some protein sources are also high in fat, cholesterol and calories, such as: beef, whole milk products, eggs, poultry with skin, cheese and nuts.

The best sources of protein are low-fat foods, including fish, poultry without skin, skim or low-fat milk products and tofu. Whole grains, vegetables and especially legumes (dried beans, peas and lentils) also contain some protein.

Unless you are a very strict vegetarian, you probably get adequate protein with a balanced diet. If you are a strict vegetarian, a nutritionist can analyze your present diet to make sure you're getting adequate amounts of protein.

Carbohydrates: energy

Total carbohydrates are made up of simple sugars, complex carbohydrates, and fiber.

Simple carbohydrates. Sources of simple carbohydrates include: table sugar, candies and other sweets, sodas and bakery goods. These foods contain little or no vitamins and minerals. They provide empty calories, i.e., calories that supply no nutrients and should therefore be minimized.

Fruits and some vegetables contain sugar naturally, and they also provide other nutrients, so they are valuable to a healthy diet. The sugar in simple carbohydrates is in a form that is absorbed quickly by the body, as opposed to the slower-digesting complex carbohydrates.

Complex carbohydrates. These carbohydrates contain many essential nutrients and are the body's most effective source of energy. They are very low in fat and should be the primary source of calories. It is recommended that 50% to 65% of total daily calories come from nutrient-dense carbohydrates. Foods high in complex carbohydrates include:

- breads and cereals
- dried beans, peas, and lentils
- potatoes and other starchy vegetables
- pasta
- rice and other grain products

Dietary Fiber. The typical American diet is much too low in fiber. The American Cancer Society recommends 20 - 30 grams of fiber daily. The average American consumes only 7 - 8 grams of fiber daily.

Dietary fiber is a term used to describe parts of plant foods which are generally not digestible by humans. By increasing your intake of foods containing complex carbohydrates, you will add dietary fiber to your diet.

There are two main types of fiber: soluble and insoluble. Soluble fiber may help lower blood cholesterol and control blood sugar. Soluble fiber is found in oats, beans, carrots, apples and oranges. Insoluble fiber helps to move food through the body quickly and protect against colorectal cancer. Insoluble fiber is found in wheat bran and whole grains. Because both types of fiber have different functions for improving health, a variety of foods with fiber should be included in your diet.

Although fruits and vegetables are not considered complex carbohydrates, they do have significant amounts of nutrients and fiber. Thus, a diet rich in whole grains, breads, cereals, fruits and vegetables will provide optimal amounts of nutrients, fiber and energy.

Diabetic food exchanges

"Exchanges," as listed on the last line of the nutrition analysis, are based on the meal planning system recommended by the American Diabetes Association.

A well-balanced and carefully controlled diet is essential for those with diabetes. Most use the food exchange system to plan meals. Foods are grouped into the various exchange lists according to their similarities in calories, carbohydrate, protein and fat content, which influence how they are utilized by the body. Although carbohydrates have the largest influence on blood sugar levels, protein and fat also contribute calories and influence the rates of digestion, so they are important to the overall plan.

Even for those without diabetes, the food exchanges which are listed can give useful information about portion size and the balance you are getting between protein and simple and complex carbohydrates, as explained below.

One meat exchange is equivalent to approximately 7 grams of protein and 3 grams of fat. One bread (starch) exchange contains approximately 15 grams of carbohydrate and 3 grams of protein. Starchy vegetables (potatoes, corn, beans, etc.) are counted as bread (starch) exchanges rather than vegetable exchanges. Vegetable exchanges have less starch (5 grams of complex carbohydrate and 2 grams of protein) and lots of fiber. A fruit exchange contains approximately 15 grams of more easily digested (simple) carbohydrate. A milk exchange contains 12 grams of carbohydrate, 8 grams of protein, and only a trace of fat, assuming skim milk is used. A fat exchange represents 5 grams of fat.

Some diabetic exchange lists use separate categories for lean, medium-fat, and high-fat meats. The computerized system used for the *Healthy Dining* analysis uses the lean meat category which assumes approximately 7 grams of protein and 3 grams of fat per meat exchange. In most entrees included in the book, the meat is very lean and the total fat from the meat is lower than the 3 grams of fat per meat exchange normally assumed. In these cases we have designated the meat exchanges as "(extra lean)," which indicates that the meat exchange contains less fat than the assumed standard of 3 grams of fat per meat exchange. Any added fat from additional ingredients (e.g., butter or oil used in preparation, sauces, spreads, etc.) is counted as separate fat exchanges. This means that the fat exchanges reflect additional fat added to the meat.

In many entrees shown in this book, extra fat (often unsaturated) is added, but with the very lean meat, the total grams of fat still comes out very low. So you don't necessarily need to shy away from a selection that shows fat exchanges. Looking at the grams of fat probably gives better information about the overall fat content.

The food exchanges used by some weight loss programs use an exchange system which is similar to the diabetic food exchange system. A dietitian can help you interpret these numbers to meet your particular dietary needs.

CHAPTER 8

Additional Tips for Healthy Dining

Here are some additional dining tips, adapted from "Eating Better When Eating Out," from the USDA Human Nutrition Information Service:

Appetizers: Enjoy raw vegetables dipped in salsa or low-calorie dressing, fruit or steamed seafood. Limit rich sauces, dips and batter-fried foods.

Soups: Choose broth or tomato-based soups rather than creamed soups. Lentil, bean and split pea soups are high in fiber. Most soups are high in sodium.

Breads: Bread supplies complex carbohydrates, vitamins, and minerals. Whole grain breads provide fiber. Watch out for breads with added fat or sugar such as croissants, biscuits, cornbread, muffins (e.g., bran, corn, blueberry) and sweet rolls. Use toppings (butter, cream cheese and margarine) very sparingly.

Vegetables and Salads: Plain vegetables are high in fiber and nutrients and very low in calories, fat and sodium. However, butter, margarine and sauces increase calories, fat, cholesterol and sodium considerably. Look for vegetables seasoned with lemon, herbs or spices rather than fat and salt. Remember -- salad dressings and toppings can add a lot of calories, fat and sodium.

Watch out for prepared salads that contain mayonnaise, salad dressing or oil, such as macaroni salad, potato salad, creamy coleslaw, tuna and chicken salad, and marinated vegetables. Some pasta salads are made with large amounts of oily dressing.

Main Entrees: Ask how meals are prepared and what ingredients are used. Is the fish or chicken broiled with butter or other fat? Is it served with a sauce? How large is the portion? Are vegetables fresh or canned, buttered or creamed?

Fish or poultry that is broiled, grilled, baked, steamed or poached is a good choice. However, entrees are often basted with large amounts of fat. Ask to have your entree prepared without added fat, and that chicken be prepared without skin (or remove the skin before eating). Request that lemon juice, wine or only a small amount of fat be used and that no salt be added.

Watch out for menu selections termed "light fare" or "light." "Light" may or may not mean lower in fat and calories. We have found restaurants in which "On the Light Side" means anything from smaller portions to lower prices!

Choose dishes flavored with herbs and spices rather than rich sauces, gravies, or dressings. If that's not an option, ask for gravies, sour cream, sauces, and other toppings to be served on the side and use sparingly. Limit your use of soy sauce, steak sauce, catsup, mustard, pickles and other condiments to help control sodium.

Portions are often very large. Ask for a take-home bag and eat the remaining portion the next day. Or share an entree with a friend and get an extra appetizer.

Many stir-fried entrees are prepared with very little oil, while some are prepared with too much. Request that yours to be prepared with very little.

Pizza can be a low-fat, nutritious choice if you order yours with half the cheese and only vegetable toppings.

Sandwiches can be an excellent choice if you choose lean deli meats such as turkey or ham (but watch portion size!) instead of higher fat cold cuts, such as bologna or salami. Choose whole grain breads and go easy on or avoid oil, butter and mayonnaise.

Desserts: Fruits are great! Sherbet, sorbet and frozen yogurt are much lower in fat than ice cream. If temptation gets to you -- share the dessert with a dinner partner.

Words that signal _high fat_ include:

buttered or buttery	creamed or creamy	rich
scalloped	fried	breaded
fritters	tempura	croquettes
crispy	with gravy	in cheese sauce
Hollandaise	au gratin	à la king
Béarnaise	Alfredo	Newburg

Words that signal _high sodium_ include:

smoked	barbecued	pickled
broth	soy sauce	teriyaki
creole sauce	marinated	cocktail sauce
tomato base	Parmesan	mustard sauce

Appendix:
Analysis Methods and Accuracy

How was the nutrition analysis done?

We used recipes supplied by the restaurant and performed a computerized nutritional analysis with the Nutritionist IV Computer program developed by N-Squared Computing in Oregon. Research shows the Nutritionist IV Program to be one of the most current and reliable nutrition analysis programs available. It uses the U.S. Department of Agriculture (USDA) data base. We regularly update our program with new data values published by the USDA. If values for recipe ingredients were not available from the USDA data base, we contacted the manufacturer for nutritional information. If the manufacturer did not have nutritional information, we closely matched ingredients to another product with nutritional information.

The data were rounded to the nearest whole number, except for diabetic exchanges, which were rounded to the nearest ¼ exchange unit. The numbers coming from the USDA data base and the computer analysis imply a high degree of accuracy. In reality, the USDA found that nutritional values of foods can vary between similar food samples by as much as 20%, and the numbers coming from their measurements represent their average data. Therefore it is important to note that the numerical values for the selected menu items published in this book are approximations only.

Notes about accuracy

The most accurate method to obtain nutritional information is a chemical analysis performed in a professional laboratory. That is, in fact, how the USDA obtained the information for their data base. It is very expensive (over $1,000 per item) and time-consuming, and therefore unrealistic for this project. Every effort was made to ensure accurate information from the computerized analysis and the USDA data base.

Two main obstacles were encountered with the computerized analysis. First, how much marinade do meats actually absorb, and second, how much oil is absorbed in flash-frying (a method commonly used in Chinese foods)? After numerous conversations with experts throughout the U.S., we found that there has been very little research in these areas. As recommended by nutritionists at the USDA and the Human Nutrition Information Service, we assumed that ¼ to ½ oz. of marinade per 8 oz. of meat was absorbed, depending on the amount of marinading time, and that very little oil (1 teaspoon/6 oz. meat) was absorbed with flash-frying.

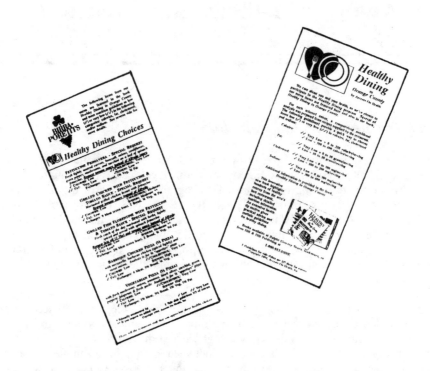

Healthy Dining menus for customer convenience.

We encourage the restaurants to pass out *Healthy Dining* menus along with their regular menus. These *Healthy Dining* menus are condensed versions of the book pages. Some restaurants, however, do not automatically provide them -- *you must request the Healthy Dining menus*. And please do! The more that restaurants hear customers asking for specific nutrition information and ordering "Special Requests," the more they will recognize how important healthy dining is to many people.

If nutrition information is important to you, if you want to have the choice to "order healthy," please request *Healthy Dining* menus in the restaurants and let them know that you appreciate the healthy menu choices.

Part II
Healthy Dining Menus

Arranged alphabetically
Also see index at back, arranged by type of cuisine, location, and alphabetically

Summary of check mark system:

ENTREE GUIDELINES†

Calories	✓✓	Very Low = 0 to 350 calories/entree
	✓	Low = 350 to 600 calories/entree
Fat	✓✓	Very Low = 0 to 10 grams (g)/entree
	✓	Low = 10 to 20 grams (g)/entree
Cholesterol	✓✓	Very Low = 0 to 75 milligrams (mg)/entree
	✓	Low = 75 to 150 milligrams (mg)/entree
Sodium	✓✓	Very Low = 0 to 300 milligrams (mg)/entree
	✓	Low = 300 to 600 milligrams (mg)/entree

Footnotes
* Primarily unsaturated fat
** If you request no added salt
† Side dish guidelines are
1/3 of entree guidelines

Price Range Symbol
$ Average entree under $10
$$ Average entree $10 - $20
$$$ Average entree over $20

Special Request - modification of the usual restaurant recipe or preparation method. You must ask for the "Special Request" to make it correspond to the published nutrition information.

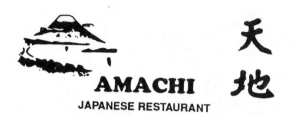

AMACHI 天地
JAPANESE RESTAURANT

Amachi Japanese Restaurant has one of the finest sushi bars in Orange County. You'll also enjoy the relaxing environment of our dining room, the tempting sushi roll specials, and a wide variety of Japanese dishes like teriyaki, tempura, and sukiyaki. Come join us for a pleasant, delicious taste of Japan and a memorable dining experience. $

Amachi Japanese Restaurant
2675 Irvine Ave., Costa Mesa, CA 92627   (714) 645-5518

SASHIMI AND CALIFORNIA ROLL
A mix of seafood, avocado, and rice for a great California taste!
✓ CALORIES: Low (407)   ✓✓ CHOLESTEROL: Very Low (66 mg)
✓✓ FAT: Very Low* (6 g)   SODIUM: Moderate (710 mg) **
Exchanges: 3¼ Meat (extra lean), 2¾ Bread, ½ Veg, ½ Fat

NIGIRI SUSHI AND CUCUMBER ROLL
Delicious fish, cucumber, and rice combination.
✓ CALORIES: Low (451)   ✓✓ CHOLESTEROL: Very Low (43 mg)
✓✓ FAT: Very Low* (4 g)   ✓ SODIUM: Low (361 mg) **
Exchanges: 2 Meat (extra lean), 4½ Bread, ½ Veg, ¼ Fat

RAINBOW ROLL
with tuna, white fish, yellowtail, salmon, shrimp, and rice.
✓✓ CALORIES: Very Low (270)   ✓✓ CHOLESTEROL: Very Low (40 mg)
✓✓ FAT: Very Low* (3 g)   ✓✓ SODIUM: Very Low (224 mg) **
Exchanges: 1½ Meat, 2½ Bread

SALMON TERIYAKI
Broiled salmon with teriyaki sauce. Served with steamed rice (not included in analysis).
✓✓ CALORIES: Very Low (343)   ✓ CHOLESTEROL: Low (106 mg)
✓ FAT: Low* (12 g)   SODIUM: High (1114 mg)
Exchanges: 5 Meat, ¾ Bread

YOSENABE
Delicious fish & seafood soup, with cabbage, tofu, onions, sake, udon noodles, and more.
✓ CALORIES: Low (426)   ✓✓ CHOLESTEROL: Very Low (59 mg)
✓✓ FAT: Very Low* (7 g)   SODIUM: High (1749 mg)
Exchanges: 4½ Meat (extra lean), 3¼ Bread, 1½ Veg, 1½ Fat

† Side dish guidelines are 1/3 of entree guidelines

✓ Low   ✓✓ Very Low

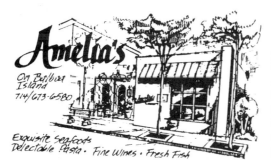

Exquisite Seafoods
Delectable Pasta · Fine Wines · Fresh Fish

For 35 years, Amelia's Seafood & Italian Restaurant has been serving the Newport Beach residents and visitors alike, who cherish the finest in delicious seafood and delectable pasta. This cozy European restaurant is tucked away amongst the quaint shops on Balboa Island's Main Street, and is Orange County's oldest family-owned restaurant at the same location. $$

Amelia's 311 Marine Ave., Balboa Island, Newport Beach, CA 92662   (714) 673-6580

FRESH FISH WITH TOMATOES AND BASIL GARNISH
Served with steamed vegetables (included in analysis) and Pasta with Marinara Sauce (see below). Analysis is for cod; other fish similar.
✓✓ CALORIES: Very Low (266)   ✓✓ CHOLESTEROL: Very Low (61 mg)
✓ FAT: Low* (15 g)   ✓✓ SODIUM: Very Low (96 mg) **
Exchanges: 2 Meat (extra lean), 1¼ Veg, 2¾ Fat

CHICKEN BREAST WITH ARTICHOKES AND MUSHROOMS
Served with steamed vegetables (included in analysis) and Pasta with Marinara Sauce (see below).
✓ CALORIES: Low (504)   ✓ CHOLESTEROL: Low (130 mg)
✓ FAT: Low (15 g)   ✓ SODIUM: Low (347 mg) **
Exchanges: 6¾ Meat (extra lean), 6½ Veg, 1¾ Fat

LASAGNA PRIMAVERA
✓ CALORIES: Low (448)   ✓ CHOLESTEROL: Low (99 mg)
✓ FAT: Low (11 g)   SODIUM: Moderate (632 mg) **
Exchanges: 1 Meat, 3¼ Bread, 2¼ Veg, ¼ Milk, ¾ Fat

ANGEL HAIR PASTA WITH TOMATOES AND BASIL - SPECIAL REQUEST
Request less oil (1 Tbs).
✓ CALORIES: Low (544)   ✓✓ CHOLESTEROL: None (0 mg)
✓ FAT: Low* (16 g)   ✓✓ SODIUM: Very Low (14 mg) **
Exchanges: 5¼ Bread, 1 Veg, 2¾ Fat

FRESH FISH SAMPLER PLATE
Served with steamed vegetables (included in analysis) and Pasta with Marinara Sauce (see below).
✓✓ CALORIES: Very Low (312)   ✓ CHOLESTEROL: Low (99 mg)
✓ FAT: Low (13 g)   ✓✓ SODIUM: Very Low (136 mg) **
Exchanges: 4¾ Meat (extra lean), ¾ Veg, ¾ Fat

PASTA WITH MARINARA SAUCE†
✓✓ CALORIES: Very Low (110)   ✓✓ CHOLESTEROL: None (0 mg)
✓✓ FAT: Very Low* (1 g)   ✓✓ SODIUM: Very Low (60 mg) **
Exchanges: 1¼ Bread, ¼ Veg

---

* Primarily unsaturated fat
** If you request no added salt

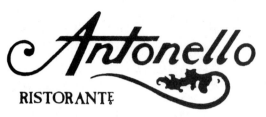

Antonello Ristorante

South Coast Plaza Village
1611 Sunflower Ave.
Santa Ana, CA 92704   (714) 751-7153

Growing up in the foothills of Italy meant fresh foods, simple meals and the everyday passion of Italian living. At Antonello's, this same adventure of the heart and authentic country food are affectionately prepared for all.

"La Cucina Leggera" is the theme of our new menu and recipes. The items are hearty and full flavored, created with healthy ingredients, and can be prepared with less oil and salt if requested to meet your special needs. $$

BRODO DI POLLO E PASTINA†
Very delicate consomme' of spring chicken with pastina.
✓ CALORIES: Low (127)   ✓✓ CHOLESTEROL: Very Low (11 mg)
✓✓ FAT: Very Low (2 g)   SODIUM: Moderate (661 mg) **
Exchanges: 1¼ Bread, ¼ Veg

BRANZINO IN GUAZETTO
Sea bass cooked in tomatoes, oregano and white wine.
✓ CALORIES: Low (468)   ✓ CHOLESTEROL: Low (94 mg)
✓ FAT: Low* (20 g)   ✓✓ SODIUM: Very Low (247 mg) **
Exchanges: 4 Meat (extra lean), ¼ Bread, 2½ Veg, 2¾ Fat

FETTUCCINE PRIMAVERA
A vegetarian creation of homemade fettuccine with garden fresh vegetables sauteed in extra virgin olive oil, basil and garlic.
✓ CALORIES: Low (367)   ✓✓ CHOLESTEROL: Very Low (56 mg)
✓✓ FAT: Very Low* (9 g)   ✓ SODIUM: Low (324 mg) **
Exchanges: 3½ Bread, 1¼ Veg, 1¼ Fat

FUSILI AI FILETTI DI POMODORO
Corkscrew pasta with fresh tomato fillets, garlic and basil sauce.
✓ CALORIES: Low (468)   ✓✓ CHOLESTEROL: None (0 mg)
✓ FAT: Low* (16 g)   ✓✓ SODIUM: Very Low (46 mg) **
Exchanges: 3¼ Bread, 4 Veg, 2¾ Fat

RIGATONI DEL BARONE
Large tubes of pasta with strips of chicken and broccoli sauteed with chopped onion, bay leaves, white wine and tomato sauce.
✓ CALORIES: Low (516)   ✓ CHOLESTEROL: Low (121 mg)
✓✓ FAT: Very Low (9 g)   SODIUM: High (1080 mg)
Exchanges: 3½ Meat (extra lean), 2¾ Bread, 6 Veg, 1 Fat

LINGUINE ALLE VONGOLE
Linguine with fresh clams and white sauce.
✓ CALORIES: Low (480)   ✓✓ CHOLESTEROL: Very Low (39 mg)
✓ FAT: Low* (17 g)   SODIUM: Moderate (651 mg) **
Exchanges: 2½ Meat (extra lean), 2¾ Bread, ½ Veg, 2¾ Fat

† Side dish guidelines are 1/3 of entree guidelines

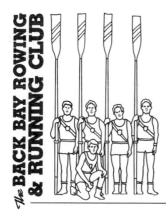

The Back Bay Rowing & Running Club

In keeping with our tradition of physical fitness, The BBR&RC Restaurant strives to serve the finest and freshest foods possible. Our soups and chili are free of preservatives. Our eggs are fresh. Our tuna is packed in water. We don't add sulphites or MSG to anything, and our salad bar filled with fresh produce was chosen "Best Salad Bar of the Year" for 7 years in a row by Orange County Magazine. $

The Back Bay Rowing & Running Club Restaurant
South Coast Plaza Mall, 3333 Bristol Street
Costa Mesa, CA 92626   (714) 641-0118

FISH TACOS
Orange roughy and hoki grilled in herbed salsa and stuffed into steamed corn tortillas with fresh black beans & napa cabbage, and served with guacamole. Soup and bread not included in analysis.
- ✓ CALORIES: Low (490)
- ✓✓ CHOLESTEROL: Very Low (17 mg)
- ✓ FAT: Low (17 g)
- ✓ SODIUM: Low (588 mg) **

Exchanges: 1¼ Meat (extra lean), 3¾ Bread, 1 Veg, 3 Fat

ROUGHY CLUB SANDWICH - SPECIAL REQUEST
Orange roughy lightly seasoned and grilled, served atop a fresh chunky avocado salsa, with shredded lettuce on a fresh sourdough roll. Request less butter (1 tsp). Cole slaw not included in analysis.
- ✓ CALORIES: Low (489)
- ✓✓ CHOLESTEROL: Very Low (28 mg)
- ✓ FAT: Low (16 g)
- SODIUM: High (1084 mg)

Exchanges: 1¾ Meat (extra lean), 3 Bread, ¼ Veg, ½ Fruit, 3 Fat

WHOLE GRAIN VEGETARIAN BURGER - SPECIAL REQUEST
Grilled and served on a sesame bun with lettuce, tomato, red onions, and slices of pickle. Request savory dressing on the side (not included in analysis).
- ✓ CALORIES: Low (594)
- ✓✓ CHOLESTEROL: None (0 mg)
- ✓✓ FAT: Very Low* (7 g)
- SODIUM: High (1018 mg)

Exchanges: 7 Bread, ½ Fruit, 1¼ Fat

TURKEY BURGER - SPECIAL REQUEST
Grilled and served on a sesame bun with lettuce, tomato, red onions, and slices of pickle. Request savory dressing on the side (not included in analysis).
- ✓ CALORIES: Low (529)
- ✓✓ CHOLESTEROL: Very Low (71 mg)
- ✓ FAT: Low (20 g)
- SODIUM: Moderate (704 mg) **

Exchanges: 3½ Meat, 3 Bread, ½ Fruit, 1½ Fat

RECOMMENDED SALAD BAR ITEMS
✓✓ Very Low   *Each ¼ cup serving of raw vegetables and fruits listed below contains less than 40 calories, less than 30 mg sodium, and no fat or cholesterol.*

Alfalfa Sprouts	Lettuce	Red Peppers	Strawberries	Pineapple
Celery	Mushrooms	Red Onions	Melons	Berries
Carrots	Spinach		Orange Slices	Thai Yum Melon

✓ Low fat, Very Low cholesterol *Each ¼ cup serving of the following has less than 60 calories, less than 3 g fat and less than 10 mg cholesterol.*

Corn Pepper Relish	Black Bean Salad	Beets in Rice Vinegar	Salsa
Red Potato Salad	Dilled Carrots	Rice Noodles with Cilantro	

* Primarily unsaturated fat
** If you request no added salt

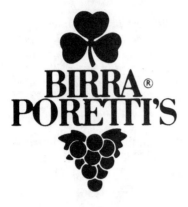

Birraporetti's -- "A Great Italian Restaurant...A Heck of an Irish Bar." The best of both worlds! Join us for an elegant dinner before an evening at the theatre, a swinging Monday night with the sounds of the big band era, or a Sunday evening for live jazz. The classy decor of the restaurant, from its high ceilings to its mahogany wood, provides the perfect ambiance for a wedding reception or a private party. So whether you're in the mood for a romantic evening, a business luncheon or dinner, or a rip-roarin' night out on the town, Birraporetti's is the hottest spot to meet in Orange County. $$

Birraporetti's   3333 S. Bristol, Costa Mesa, CA 92626   (714) 850-9090

FETTUCCINE PRIMAVERA - SPECIAL REQUEST
Fresh lightly sauteed carrots, broccoli, onions, cauliflower, green pepper, mushrooms, and zucchini on a bed of spinach fettuccine. Request tomato sauce instead of Alfredo sauce.

✓ CALORIES: Low (385)   ✓✓ CHOLESTEROL: Very Low (1 mg)
✓✓ FAT: Very Low (5 g)   ✓ SODIUM: Low (489 mg) **
Exchanges: 3¾ Bread, 1¾ Veg, ¾ Fat

GRILLED CHICKEN WITH FETTUCCINE & TOMATO SAUCE - SPECIAL REQUEST
Marinated grilled chicken breast with fettuccine. Request tomato sauce instead of Alfredo.

✓ CALORIES: Low (550)   CHOLESTEROL: Moderate (174 mg)
✓ FAT: Low (11 g)   SODIUM: Moderate (646 mg) **
Exchanges: 9 Meat (extra lean), 2 Bread, ¾ Veg, ¾ Fat

GRILLED FISH FLORENTINE WITH FETTUCCINE & TOMATO SAUCE - SPECIAL REQUEST
Fresh catch of the day marinated with herbs, lightly spiced and served with spinach fettuccine. Request less oil (1 Tbs) and tomato sauce instead of Alfredo.

✓ CALORIES: Low (486)   ✓✓ CHOLESTEROL: Very Low (45 mg)
✓ FAT: Low* (19 g)   SODIUM: Moderate (733 mg) **
Exchanges: 2¾ Meat (extra lean), 2 Bread, ¾ Veg, 3¼ Fat

BARBEQUE CHICKEN PIZZA (½ PIZZA)
with mozzarella, barbecue chicken (spiced lightly) and sweet onions.
Analysis is for ½ "appetizer" pizza.

✓ CALORIES: Low (536)   ✓✓ CHOLESTEROL: Very Low (75 mg)
✓ FAT: Low (15 g)   SODIUM: High (1007 mg)
Exchanges: 4 Meat, 3¾ Bread, ¼ Veg, 1 Fat

VEGETARIAN PIZZA (½ PIZZA)
with fresh mushrooms, onions, tomatoes, black olives, zucchini, green peppers, jalapenos and fresh garlic. Analysis is for ½ "appetizer" pizza.

✓ CALORIES: Low (504)   ✓✓ CHOLESTEROL: Very Low (32 mg)
✓ FAT: Low (16 g)   SODIUM: High (1104 mg)
Exchanges: 1¾ Meat, 3½ Bread, 1¾ Veg, 1¼ Fat

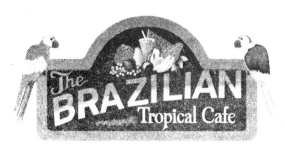

Experience authentic Brazilian cuisine made with only the finest, freshest ingredients. Conveniently located in the Atrium Court at Fashion Island, The Brazilian Tropical Cafe offers a new concept in fast gourmet food, with large, balanced portions at reasonable prices. The unique menu features a variety of festive crepes and a selection of traditional Brazilian entrees, all beautifully prepared and served promptly by our friendly staff.
$

The Brazilian Tropical Cafe
401 Newport Center Drive #A-106, Newport Beach, CA 92660 (714) 720-1522

VEGGIE BROCHETTE
Mixed vegetable brochettes with brown rice, beans and green salad.
We recommend fat-free dressing (not included in analysis).
✓✓ CALORIES: Very Low (305)   ✓✓ CHOLESTEROL: None (0 mg)
✓✓ FAT: Very Low* (3 g)   ✓ SODIUM: Low (425 mg) **
Exchanges: ¼ Meat, 3 Bread, 2½ Veg

RIO MEAL WITH CHICKEN (SMALL SIZE)
Grilled chicken served with veggies, brown rice and your choice of pinto or black beans.
✓✓ CALORIES: Very Low (308)   ✓✓ CHOLESTEROL: Very Low (65 mg)
✓✓ FAT: Very Low (4 g)   ✓ SODIUM: Low (341 mg) **
Exchanges: 3½ Meat (extra lean), 2¼ Bread, ½ Veg

LITE CREPE (REGULAR SIZE)
Broiled chicken, alfalfa sprouts, papaya salsa, corn, bell pepper and yogurt dressing.
✓✓ CALORIES: Very Low (291)   ✓ CHOLESTEROL: Low (98 mg)
✓✓ FAT: Very Low (5 g)   ✓✓ SODIUM: Very Low (119 mg) **
Exchanges: 3½ Meat (extra lean), ¾ Bread, ¾ Veg, ¼ Milk, ½ Fruit, ¼ Fat

SPICY BAHIA CREPE (REGULAR SIZE)
Sautéed shrimp or chicken in spicy Bahia sauce (tomato & mushroom) with rice. Analysis is for shrimp.
✓✓ CALORIES: Very Low (332)   CHOLESTEROL: Moderate (167 mg)
✓✓ FAT: Very Low* (4 g)   SODIUM: Moderate (611 mg) **
Exchanges: 1½ Meat (extra lean), 2¾ Bread, 1¼ Veg, ¼ Fat

GRILLED CHICKEN BREAST
Marinated chicken breast with fresh herbs, brown rice, veggies & beans. Bahia Sauce shown below.
✓ CALORIES: Low (483)   ✓ CHOLESTEROL: Low (108 mg)
✓✓ FAT: Very Low (8 g)   SODIUM: Moderate (605 mg) **
Exchanges: 6 Meat (extra lean), 3 Bread, 1 Veg, ¼ Fat

GRILLED FRESH FISH
with brown rice, veggies, & black or pinto beans. Bahia Sauce shown below.
Analysis for mahi mahi; other fish similar.
✓ CALORIES: Low (432)   ✓ CHOLESTEROL: Low (93 mg)
✓✓ FAT: Very Low* (10 g)   SODIUM: Moderate (605 mg) **
Exchanges: 2¼ Meat (extra lean), 3 Bread, 1 Veg, 1½ Fat

BAHIA SAUCE *(2 oz)* 17 calories, ½ g fat, 1 mg cholesterol, 171 mg sodium.

---

* Primarily unsaturated fat
** If you request no added salt

Healthy Dining in Orange County   **51**

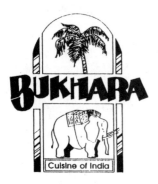

Bukhara is the ancient city where the Mughlai style of Indian cooking originated. Indian cuisine is a delicate blend of subtle flavors as varied as India's climate and as elegant as its culture. Let us introduce you to these exotic dishes. You can even observe the chef prepare Tandoori specialties behind the glass window. Please join us for a distinctive dining experience at Bukhara. $$

Bukhara Cuisine of India

7594 Edinger Ave, Huntington Beach 92647   (714) 842-3171
16260 Ventura Blvd, Encino, CA 91436   (818) 906-8472

FISH TIKKA KABAB (½ SERVING)
Fish pieces marinated lightly in garlic & herbs, served with tomatoes. Analysis is for ½ full plate.
✓✓ CALORIES: Very Low (244)   ✓✓ CHOLESTEROL: Very Low (67 mg)
✓✓ FAT: Very Low* (9 g)   ✓✓ SODIUM: Very Low (165 mg) **
Exchanges: 3¾ Meat, ½ Veg, ¼ Fat

KARAHI CHICKEN (½ SERVING)
Chicken cooked in juice of garlic, ginger and tomatoes in a karahi (special pan). Analysis is for ½ full plate.
✓✓ CALORIES: Very Low (248)   ✓ CHOLESTEROL: Low (87 mg)
✓ FAT: Low (11 g)   ✓✓ SODIUM: Very Low (88 mg) **
Exchanges: 4½ Meat (extra lean), ¼ Veg, 1¼ Fat

CHICKEN TIKKA MASALA (½ SERVING)
Boneless tandoori chicken delicately cooked in a gravy of tomatoes, cream, onions and spices. Analysis is for ½ full plate.
✓ CALORIES: Low (402)   ✓ CHOLESTEROL: Low (140 mg)
✓ FAT: Low (15 g)   ✓ SODIUM: Low (475 mg) **
Exchanges: 6¾ Meat (extra lean), 2¼ Veg, 1¾ Fat

VEGETABLE PILLAU (½ SERVING)
Basmati rice cooked with vegetables & nuts with aroma of saffron. Analysis is for ½ full plate.
✓ CALORIES: Low (457)   ✓✓ CHOLESTEROL: None (0 mg)
✓✓ FAT: Very Low* (9 g)   ✓✓ SODIUM: Very Low (58 mg) **
Exchanges: 5 Bread, 1¼ Veg, 1½ Fat

ALOO GOBI (½ SERVING)
Cauliflower and potatoes sauteed in mild herbs and spices. Analysis is for ½ full plate.
✓✓ CALORIES: Very Low (201)   ✓✓ CHOLESTEROL: None (0 mg)
✓✓ FAT: Very Low (8 g)   ✓✓ SODIUM: Very Low (30 mg) **
Exchanges: 1½ Bread, 1 Veg, 1¼ Fat

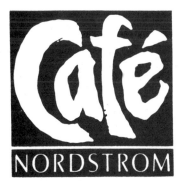

Cafe Nordstrom

Cafe Nordstrom offers a wide selection of breakfast items, hot and cold sandwiches, specialty salads and freshly baked pastries to hungry shoppers. Especially popular with our lunch crowd is our Blue Plate Souper which features a bowl of soup, green salad and a half sandwich. At Cafe Nordstrom we take pride in the freshness and quality of our food. $

South Coast Plaza: 3333 Bristol Street, Costa Mesa, CA 92626   (714) 549-8300
Brea Mall: 500 Brea Mall Way, Brea, CA 92521   (714) 529-0123
Montclair: 5015 Montclair Plaza Lane, Montclair, CA 91762   (909) 625-0821
Main Place (Santa Ana): 2820 North Main, Santa Ana, CA 92701   (714) 972-2020
Tyler Mall (Riverside): 3601 Tyler Street, Riverside, CA 92503   (909) 351-3170

THE ORIGINAL GARDEN BURGER
Totally meatless, low-fat, soy-free and very delicious! Served on a squaw roll with lettuce, tomato, sprouts, a slice of onion, and served with tossed green salad.
- ✓ CALORIES. Low (382)
- ✓✓ CHOLESTEROL: Very Low (18 mg)
- ✓✓ FAT: Very Low (10 g)
- SODIUM: Moderate (623 mg)**

Exchanges: ½ Meat, 3½ Bread, ½ Veg, 1¾ Fat

VEGETARIAN CHILI WITH BEANS
Served with Foccacia bread (not included in analysis).
- ✓✓ CALORIES: Very Low (300)
- ✓✓ CHOLESTEROL: Very Low (30 mg)
- ✓ FAT: Low (13 g)
- SODIUM: High (1100 mg)

Exchanges: 1 Meat, 2½ Bread, ¼ Veg, 1¼ Fat

BREAST OF TURKEY SANDWICH - SPECIAL REQUEST
Request no mayonnaise.
- ✓✓ CALORIES: Very Low (268)
- ✓ CHOLESTEROL: Low (86 mg)
- ✓✓ FAT: Very Low (3 g)
- SODIUM: High (1712 mg)

Exchanges: 3½ Meat (extra lean), 1½ Bread, ¼ Veg, ½ Fat

GRILLED CHICKEN CHOP SALAD - SPECIAL REQUEST
Grilled chicken breast cut into strips, mixed together with crisp mixed greens, grated mozzarella cheese, fresh basil and sundried tomatoes, then chopped into delicate morsels. Request ½ portion of cheese & low-cal dressing or dressing on the side (dressing not included in analysis).
- ✓ CALORIES: Low (395)
- ✓ CHOLESTEROL: Low (119 mg)
- ✓ FAT: Low (14 g)
- ✓✓ SODIUM: Very Low (276 mg) **

Exchanges: 5¼ Meat, 1 Veg, 1½ Fat

BAR-B-QUE CHICKEN SALAD - SPECIAL REQUEST
Crisp mixed greens, topped with baked chicken breast in BBQ sauce, black beans, cheddar cheese, mozzarella cheese, tomato, and green onion with ranch dressing on the side (dressing not included in analysis). Request ½ portion of cheese.
- ✓ CALORIES: Low (515)
- ✓ CHOLESTEROL: Low (112 mg)
- ✓ FAT: Low (13 g)
- ✓ SODIUM: Low (372 mg)**

Diabetic Exchanges: 5¼ Meat, 2½ Bread, 1¼ Veg, 1 Fat

* Primarily unsaturated fat
** If you request no added salt

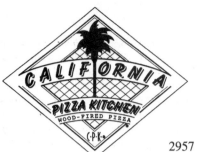

California Pizza Kitchen offers a wide range of pizzas, pastas, salads and desserts served in a bright, sleek setting. Famous for its wood-fired "California pizzas," California Pizza Kitchen has developed such imaginative fare as Barbecued Chicken, Thai Chicken and BLT pizzas. $

California Pizza Kitchen

2957 Michelson Drive, Irvine, CA 92715   (714) 975-1585
24155 Laguna Hills Mall, Laguna Hills, CA 92653   (714) 458-9600
25513 Marguerite Pkwy, Mission Viejo, CA 92692   (714) 951-5026
2800 N. Main St, Main Place Mall, Santa Ana, CA 92701   (714) 479-0604
1151 Newport Center Drive, Fashion Island, Newport Beach, CA 92660   (714) 759-5543

Any of the pizzas can be ordered cheeseless, which saves approximately 170 calories and 14 grams of fat per ½ pizza.

GRILLED TERIYAKI CHICKEN PIZZA (½ PIZZA)
with grilled chicken marinated in an orange-teriyaki sauce, red onions, scallions and sweet peppers. Analysis is for ½ pizza.
✓ CALORIES: Low (439)   ✓✓ CHOLESTEROL: Very Low (57 mg)
✓ FAT: Low (16 g)   SODIUM: High (1758 mg)
Exchanges: 2¼ Meat, 2½ Bread, ¼ Veg, 2 Fat

VEGETARIAN PIZZA (½ PIZZA)
with broccoli, onions, mushrooms, sun-dried tomatoes, grilled eggplant, fresh oregano and tomato sauce. Analysis is for ½ pizza.
✓ CALORIES: Low (452)   ✓✓ CHOLESTEROL: Very Low (41 mg)
✓ FAT: Low (18 g)   SODIUM: Moderate (946 mg) **
Exchanges: 1¼ Meat, 2½ Bread, ¾ Veg, 2½ Fat

SOUTHWESTERN BURRITO PIZZA (½ PIZZA)
with grilled chicken breast marinated in lime and herbs, Southwestern black beans, fire-roasted mild chilies, sweet white onions & cheddar cheese. Served with sour cream (not included in analysis). Analysis for ½ pizza.
✓ CALORIES: Low (494)   ✓ CHOLESTEROL: Low (83 mg)
✓ FAT: Low (20 g)   SODIUM: Moderate (936 mg) **
Exchanges: 3¼ Meat, 2½ Bread, ½ Veg, 2½ Fat

BROCCOLI SUNDRIED TOMATO FUSILLI - SPECIAL REQUEST
Corkscrew pasta with fresh broccoli, browned garlic, sun-dried tomatoes, fresh thyme and Parmesan cheese. Request no oil.
✓ CALORIES: Low (483)   ✓✓ CHOLESTEROL: Very Low (21 mg)
✓✓ FAT: Very Low (10 g)   ✓ SODIUM: Low (567 mg) **
Exchanges: 1½ Meat, 3¼ Bread, 2¼ Veg, ½ Fat

PASTA PRIMAVERA - SPECIAL REQUEST
Spaghetti with broccoli, mushrooms, tomatoes, petite peas, zucchini, yellow squash, garlic and fresh garden herbs. Request no oil.
✓✓ CALORIES: Very Low (344)   ✓✓ CHOLESTEROL: None (0 mg)
✓✓ FAT: Very Low (2 g)   SODIUM: Moderate (886 mg) **
Exchanges: 3½ Bread, 3¼ Veg

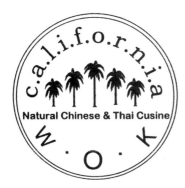

Natural Chinese & Thai Cusine

California Wok creatively captures the trend toward fresh food and Asian influence in Southern California. We emphasize the modern approach to Chinese and Thai cuisine, from the decor with dusty pink walls and black chairs, to the delicious flavors and crispness of the vegetables. We will gladly prepare any item on our menu without oil or salt upon your request. Each and every dish is prepared with tender loving care for your fullest enjoyment. After all, we are what we eat, and healthy hearts are happy hearts. $

California Wok

4466 Cerritos Avenue, Los Alamitos, CA   90720
(714) 527-0226

WOR WONTON SOUP

Dumpling soup with barbecued pork, shrimp, chicken, and mixed vegetables in thin chicken broth.

✓ CALORIES: Low (352)   ✓ CHOLESTEROL: Low (103 mg)
✓ FAT: Low (12 g)   ✓ SODIUM: Low (425 mg) **
Exchanges: 3½ Meat (extra lean), 1½ Bread, ¾ Veg, 1¼ Fat

RAINBOW CHICKEN

Slices of chicken breast stir-fried with mixed vegetables in the chef's special white wine sauce.

✓ CALORIES: Low (379)   ✓ CHOLESTEROL: Low (130 mg)
✓✓ FAT: Very Low (7 g)   ✓✓ SODIUM: Very Low (250 mg) **
Exchanges: 7 Meat (extra lean), ¾ Bread, 2¾ Veg, ¼ Fat

TEPPANYAKI VEGETABLES AND TOFU

A mixture of vegetables -- broccoli, red onions, fresh mushrooms, snow peas and bean sprouts, stir-fried with tofu and served with a delicate ginger, garlic and mustard sauce on the side (2 Tbs. included in analysis). Chicken or shrimp versions of this dish also available.

✓✓ CALORIES: Very Low (256)   ✓✓ CHOLESTEROL: Very Low (1 mg)
✓ FAT: Low* (12 g)   ✓ SODIUM: Low (553 mg) **
Exchanges: 3¼ Bread, 3½ Veg, 1¾ Fat

SHRIMP IN HOT GARLIC SAUCE

Shrimp sauteed with mixed vegetables in hot garlic sauce.

✓✓ CALORIES: Very Low (263)   CHOLESTEROL: Moderate (219 mg)
✓✓ FAT: Very Low* (7 g)   SODIUM: Moderate (649 mg) **
Exchanges: 2 Meat (extra lean), ½ Bread, 2¼ Veg, 1 Fat

LARB GAI (CHICKEN)

Chopped chicken with ground rice grain, mint leaves, lime juice and chili, served with crisp cabbage leaves.

✓ CALORIES: Low (424)   ✓ CHOLESTEROL: Low (130 mg)
✓✓ FAT: Very Low (7 g)   SODIUM: High (1064 mg)
Exchanges: 6¾ Meat (extra lean), 1¼ Bread, 2½ Veg, ¼ Fruit

---

* Primarily unsaturated fat
** If you request no added salt

THE CANNERY

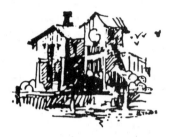

Historic landmark in Cannery Village, serving award-winning seafood, fresh fish, and eastern beef in an authentic 1930's setting, or dine outside on the waterfront deck, or upstairs in the lounge with a great harbor view, entertainment, and seafood bar. Champagne Brunch served ashore or afloat on the Cannery Cruise Boat. $$

The Cannery
3010 La Fayette Ave.
Newport Beach, CA 92663

(714) 675-5777
FAX (714) 675-2510

SEAFOOD TACOS (LUNCH ONLY) - SPECIAL REQUEST
Two soft tacos filled with seasoned grilled fresh fish, onions, cilantro, tomato & cheese. Served with refried beans, guacamole and salsa (guacamole & salsa not included in analysis). Request less cheese (1 oz) and no butter.
✓ CALORIES: Low (477)   ✓✓ CHOLESTEROL: Very Low (55 mg)
✓ FAT: Low (13 g)   SODIUM: Moderate (612 mg) **
Exchanges: 2 Meat, 3¼ Bread, 2¼ Veg, 1¾ Fat

CALIFORNIA PASTA - SPECIAL REQUEST
Fresh tomato, basil and garlic sauteed lightly, served on a bed of angel hair pasta, then topped with parmesan cheese. Request no oil.
✓ CALORIES: Low (526)   ✓✓ CHOLESTEROL: Very Low (22 mg)
✓ FAT: Low (14 g)   SODIUM: Moderate (726 mg) **
Exchanges: 1¾ Meat, 3¾ Bread, 3½ Veg, 1¼ Fat

FRESH HALIBUT - SPECIAL REQUEST
Request no butter. Analysis includes rice pilaf and steamed vegetables.
✓ CALORIES: Low (494)   ✓ CHOLESTEROL: Low (81 mg)
✓✓ FAT: Very Low* (10 g)   SODIUM: Moderate (721 mg) **
Exchanges: 4½ Meat (extra lean), 2 Bread, ¾ Veg, ¾ Fat

NEWPORT BROIL - SPECIAL REQUEST
Jumbo shrimp, fresh vegetables and slices of rose potato quickly flame broiled to perfection. Request no butter.
✓ CALORIES: Low (456)   CHOLESTEROL: Moderate (220 mg)
✓ FAT: Low* (16 g)   ✓ SODIUM: Low (327 mg) **
Exchanges: 2 Meat (extra lean), 2¼ Bread, 2½ Veg, 2¾ Fat

FRESH SWORDFISH - SPECIAL REQUEST
Request no butter. Analysis includes rice pilaf and steamed vegetables.
✓ CALORIES: Low (557)   ✓ CHOLESTEROL: Low (120 mg)
✓ FAT: Low* (15 g)   SODIUM: Moderate (837 mg) **
Exchanges: 6¼ Meat (extra lean), 2 Bread, ¾ Veg, ¾ Fat

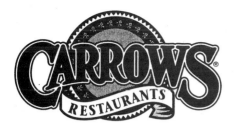

Welcome to Carrows, where food is made the old-fashioned way -- carefully prepared to order from fresh ingredients, with homestyle recipes made from scratch. From our entrees to our desserts, we'll bring back memories when folks had the time to cook food right and you couldn't wait for seconds. You'll love Carrows comfortable surroundings, friendly service and abundant portions. Of course you'll also want to save room for one of our irresistible desserts, like our "Guilt Free" No Sugar Added Apple Pie. Our bakeries (in select locations) offer fresh baked goods like muffins, cookies, and cornbread. Visit Carrows 7 days a week, from 6:00 am to 12:00 midnight (hours vary by location). $

Carrows

Locations in Anaheim, Buena Park, Fullerton, Huntington Beach, Irvine, La Habra, Laguna Hills, Mission Viejo, Newport Beach, Orange, San Clemente, and Santa Ana

---

TERIYAKI CHICKEN - SPECIAL REQUEST

A tender breast of chicken basted in teriyaki sauce and broiled to perfection. Analysis includes potato and vegetables. Request no butter on potato and vegetables. Bread not included in analysis.

✓ CALORIES: Low (598)   ✓✓ CHOLESTEROL: Very Low (75 mg)
✓✓ FAT: Very Low (7 g)   SODIUM: Moderate (791 mg) **
Exchanges: 5 Meat (extra lean), 4¾ Bread, 1 Veg, ½ Fruit, ¼ Fat

CHICKEN DELUXE SANDWICH - SPECIAL REQUEST

Lightly seasoned skinless chicken breast, topped with tomato, red onion and sprouts. Request dijon sauce on the side (not included in analysis). Request bun dry, fruit instead of fries and Catalina fat-free dressing on salad (included in analysis).

✓ CALORIES: Low (586)   ✓ CHOLESTEROL: Low (108 mg)
✓✓ FAT: Very Low (10 g)   SODIUM: High (1077 mg) **
Exchanges: 5¾ Meat (extra lean), 3 Bread, 1 Veg, 1 Fruit, ¾ Fat

FRESH VEGETABLE PLATTER - SPECIAL REQUEST

A medley of seasonal fresh vegetables & new potatoes. Request Catalina fat-free dressing instead of Hollandaise or butter (not included in analysis). Request wheat bread with no butter (included in analysis).

✓ CALORIES: Low (554)   ✓✓ CHOLESTEROL: Very Low (33 mg)
✓ FAT: Low (17 g)   SODIUM: Moderate (725 mg) **
Exchanges: 4½ Veg, 4 Bread, 3¼ Fat

GARDENBURGER - SPECIAL REQUEST

A savory, 100% meatless patty topped with lettuce, tomato, red onion and sprouts. Request dijon sauce on the side (not included in analysis). Request fruit instead of fries and Catalina fat-free dressing on salad (included in analysis).

✓ CALORIES: Low (597)   ✓✓ CHOLESTEROL: Very Low (9 mg)
✓ FAT: Low* (12 g)   SODIUM: High (1173 mg) **
Exchanges: ¾ Meat, 5 Bread, ¾ Veg, 1 Fruit, 2 Fat

BROILED SEAFOOD PLATTER

A tempting selection of Alaskan halibut, skewered shrimp and sea scallops broiled to perfection and served on rice pilaf. Analysis includes seafood and rice only.

✓ CALORIES: Low (560)   CHOLESTEROL: Moderate (255 mg)
✓ FAT: Low* (14 g)   SODIUM: High (1246 mg) **
Exchanges: 6¾ Meat (extra lean), 2¼ Bread, 1¾ Fat

* Primarily unsaturated fat
** If you request no added salt

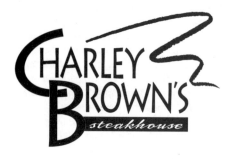

For over 30 years, Charley Brown's has been a California tradition. Enjoy savory steaks, our famous USDA Choice prime rib, fresh seafood, fresh pasta and chicken, and homemade soups, all made with the freshest ingredients. We're open daily for lunch and dinner, including our incredible Sunday Champagne Buffet Brunch. Located adjacent to Anaheim Stadium and The Arrowhead Pond, we offer free shuttle service to major events. Discover the classic flavors of Charley Brown's. $$

Charley Brown's

1751 S. State College Blvd. (corner of Katella), Anaheim, CA 92806 (714) 634-2211

FRESH SNAPPER WITH "SIMPLY LIGHT" TOPPING
Covered in a light tomato-basil vinaigrette.

✓✓ CALORIES: Very Low (309)   ✓ CHOLESTEROL: Low (82 mg)
✓ FAT: Low* (14 g)   ✓ SODIUM: Low (306 mg)**
Exchanges: 3¾ Meat (extra lean), ¼ Veg, 2¼ Fat

NORTHERN HALIBUT MONTEREY STYLE
Topped with plump Gulf shrimp, tomato, garlic & green onions, sautéed together in dry vermouth.

✓ CALORIES: Low (406)   CHOLESTEROL: Moderate (182 mg)
✓ FAT: Low (17 g)   ✓ SODIUM: Low (333 mg) **
Exchanges: 4¾ Meat (extra lean), 1 Veg, 2¼ Fat

BALSAMIC GRILLED CHICKEN
A plump, juicy breast of chicken, marinated in balsamic vinegar, olive oil, roasted garlic, thyme, rosemary and selected spices. Then it's grilled and served on a bed of freshly sautéed spinach. Very light, very delicious.

✓ CALORIES: Low (489)   CHOLESTEROL: Moderate (189 mg)
✓ FAT: Low (18 g)   SODIUM: Moderate (626 mg)**
Exchanges: 9 Meat (extra lean), 1¾ Veg, 2 Fat

FRESH SWORDFISH WITH ROASTED GARLIC & SPINACH - SPECIAL REQUEST
Topped with flavorful roasted garlic sautéed with fresh spinach and roasted red peppers. Request less butter (¼ oz).

✓✓ CALORIES: Very Low (341)   ✓ CHOLESTEROL: Low (94 mg)
✓ FAT: Low (16 g)   ✓ SODIUM: Low (525 mg)**
Exchanges: 4½ Meat (extra lean), ¾ Veg, 1½ Fat

CHAR-GRILLED VEGETABLE PASTA - SPECIAL REQUEST
We char-grill yellow squash, red peppers, zucchini, carrots, green onions and herbs, mix them with Italian olive oil and garlic and serve it up on a bed of fusilli pasta. Light and flavorful. Request less oil (¼ oz) and parmesan cheese on the side (cheese not included in analysis).

✓ CALORIES: Low (429)   ✓✓ CHOLESTEROL: None (0 mg)
✓ FAT: Low* (16 g)   ✓✓ SODIUM: Very Low (265 mg)**
Exchanges: 3¼ Bread, 2 Veg, 3 Fat

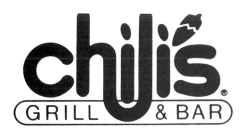

Chili's is an original -- with outstanding Southwest-style food in a casual, friendly, fun-feeling place. Come in and see why "no place else" has the food or feeling of Chili's.

And now...announcing the new "Guiltless Grill" menu items, which include low-fat and low-calorie versions of some of the restaurant's more popular offerings. All items are available to go. $

Chili's locations:

Cypress: 10643 Valley View Blvd
Foothill Ranch: 26782 Portola Pkwy
Huntington Beach: 17071 Beach Blvd
Irvine: 3745 Alton Parkway

La Palma: 40 Center Point Drive
Mission Viejo: 27407 Bellogente
Newport Beach: 3300 West Coast Hwy
Yorba Linda: 18380 Yorba Linda Blvd

GUILTLESS CHICKEN SALAD
Charbroiled chicken, mixed greens, pico de gallo, kidney beans, sprouts, green onions & our no-fat Southwest dressing.
✓✓ CALORIES: Very Low (254)   ✓ CHOLESTEROL: Low (99 mg)
✓✓ FAT: Very Low (3 g)   SODIUM: High (1547 mg)
Exchanges: 5 Meat (extra lean), 1 Bread, ½ Veg

GUILTLESS GRILLED CHICKEN SANDWICH
Charbroiled chicken with no-fat honey-mustard, lettuce, pickles & tomato. Served with fresh steamed veggies with Parmesan cheese & low-fat pasta salad (pasta salad not included in analysis).
✓ CALORIES: Low (460)   ✓ CHOLESTEROL: Low (98 mg)
✓✓ FAT: Very Low (7 g) SODIUM: High (1401 mg)
Exchanges: 5 Meat (extra lean), 2 Bread, 1 Veg, ¾ Fat

GUILTLESS GRILLED CHICKEN PLATTER
Chicken breast, charbroiled & served with rice, corn cobbette and fresh steamed veggies with Parmesan cheese.
✓ CALORIES: Low (451)   ✓ CHOLESTEROL: Low (96 mg)
✓✓ FAT: Very Low (6 g) SODIUM: Moderate (825 mg) **
Exchanges: 5 Meat (extra lean), 3¾ Bread, ¾ Veg

GUILTLESS VEGGIE PASTA
✓ CALORIES: Low (498)   ✓✓ CHOLESTEROL: Very Low (2 mg)
✓ FAT: Low (11 g)   SODIUM: High (1334 mg)
Exchanges: 4¼ Bread, 4¾ Veg, ½ Fat

GUILTLESS VEGGIE PASTA WITH CHICKEN
CALORIES: Moderate (608)   ✓ CHOLESTEROL: Low (98 mg)
✓ FAT: Low (13 g)   SODIUM: High (1456 mg)
Exchanges: 5 Meat, 4¼ Bread, 4¾ Veg, ½ Fat

LOW FAT CHOCOLATE CAKE
Delicious, rich-tasting, with only 3 grams of fat!

GUILTLESS SMOOTHIES
Orange Swirl Smoothie or Southwest Sling, with no fat and under 200 calories.

* Primarily unsaturated fat
** If you request no added salt

Healthy Dining in Orange County   **59**

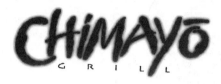

Located in Newport Beach's Fashion Island, Chimayo is restaurateur David Wilhelm's latest creation featuring Southwestern cuisine. The decor is a rich and warm blending of coastal California and Santa Fe, featuring sunset-colored walls and colorful contemporary art. A full service bar features premium tequilas, beers and wines. Patio and fireplace dining is available. Open for lunch and dinner daily. $$

Chimayo Grill

327 Newport Center Drive, Fashion Island, Newport Beach, CA 92660   (714) 640-2700

RARE AHI PEPPER STEAK
with Poblano chile sauce and vegetable medley. Corn pudding not included in analysis.
- ✓ CALORIES: Low (397)
- ✓ FAT: Low* (19 g)
- ✓✓ CHOLESTEROL: Very Low (74 mg)
- ✓✓ SODIUM: Very Low (184 mg) **

Exchanges: 3¼ Meat (extra lean), ½ Bread, 1¼ Veg, 3½ Fat

GRILLED SEAFOOD STEW
with creamy polenta, fire-roasted tortilla soup and vegetable medley.
- ✓ CALORIES: Low (486)
- ✓ FAT: Low* (15 g)
- CHOLESTEROL: Moderate (219 mg)
- SODIUM: Moderate (862 mg) **

Exchanges: 5 Meat (extra lean), 1½ Bread, 1¾ Veg, 1½ Fat

GRILLED CHICKEN - SPECIAL REQUEST
with fire roasted tortilla soup and vegetable medley. Polenta not included in analysis.
Request chicken grilled without skin.
- ✓ CALORIES: Low (593)
- FAT: Moderate (26 g)
- CHOLESTEROL: Moderate (184 mg)
- ✓ SODIUM: Low (359 mg) **

Exchanges: 9½ Meat (extra lean), ½ Bread, 1½ Veg, 3½ Fat

BBQ SALMON IN CORN HUSK
Salmon topped with Poblano pesto and corn salsa, and served with vegetable medley.
Mashed potatoes not included in analysis.
- ✓ CALORIES: Low (377)
- ✓ FAT: Low* (19 g)
- ✓ CHOLESTEROL: Low (92 mg)
- ✓ SODIUM: Low (387 mg) **

Exchanges: 4¼ Meat, ¾ Bread, 1 Veg, 1½ Fat

ANGEL HAIR PASTA WITH BASIL, TOMATOES AND GARLIC - SPECIAL REQUEST
Request less oil (½ oz) and less cheese (½ oz).
- ✓ CALORIES: Low (578)
- ✓ FAT: Low (20 g)
- ✓✓ CHOLESTEROL: Very Low (15 mg)
- ✓✓ SODIUM: Very Low (140 mg) **

Exchanges: ½ Meat, 4¼ Bread, 2¾ Veg, 3¼ Fat

* Primarily unsaturated fat
** If you request no added salt

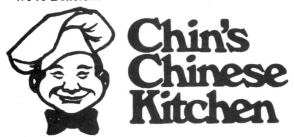

"We're Delicious"

Chin's Chinese Kitchen

Our goal is to serve the freshest, tastiest Chinese food possible. To ensure quality, we have daily deliveries from our suppliers, including trips to the market to hand pick certain produce. Each dish is cooked to order and to the customer's specifications if requested. Any addition or deletion of ingredients such as salt, sugar, MSG, garlic, starch, etc. will be made upon request. $

Chin's Chinese Kitchen

Newport Beach: 3136 W. Balboa Blvd. (on 32nd and Newport)   (714) 673-8204
Santa Ana: 124 W. MacArthur (MacMain Plaza, corner of Main St.)   (714) 546-5688
Tustin: 13771 Newport Ave (Tustin Plaza, Newport Ave & Main St.)   (714) 838-0603

SNOWPEAS WITH SHRIMP (½ SERVING)
Analysis is for ½ serving.
✓✓ CALORIES: Very Low (196)   ✓ CHOLESTEROL: Low (132 mg)
✓✓ FAT: Very Low* (8 g)   ✓ SODIUM: Low (445 mg) #
Exchanges: 1½ Meat (extra lean), ½ Bread, ½ Veg, 1¼ Fat

BROCCOLI CHICKEN (½ SERVING)
Analysis is for ½ serving.
✓✓ CALORIES: Very Low (289)   ✓ CHOLESTEROL: Low (88 mg)
✓ FAT: Low (11 g)   ✓ SODIUM: Low (398 mg) #
Exchanges: 4¾ Meat (extra lean), 1½ Veg, 1¼ Fat

CHICKEN CHOW MEIN (½ SERVING) - SPECIAL REQUEST
Request with rice instead of crunchy noodles.
Analysis includes ½ serving of chow mein and ½ cup rice.
✓ CALORIES: Low (362)   ✓ CHOLESTEROL: Low (88 mg)
✓✓ FAT: Very Low (8 g)   ✓ SODIUM: Low (388 mg) #
Exchanges: 4¾ Meat (extra lean), 1¾ Veg, ¾ Fat

MIXED VEGETABLES (½ SERVING)
Analysis is for ½ serving.
✓✓ CALORIES: Very Low (161)   ✓✓ CHOLESTEROL: Very Low (1 mg)
✓✓ FAT: Very Low (8 g)   ✓ SODIUM: Low (365 mg) #
Exchanges: ¼ Meat, ¼ Bread, 3 Veg, 1¼ Fat

* Primarily unsaturated fat
# If you request no added salt or MSG

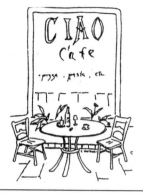

Pizzas, pastas, salads and more, all prepared fresh and healthy!

New location on beautiful Balboa Island. Dine in, take out, or call for delivery. $

Ciao
223 Marine Avenue
Balboa Island, CA 92662
(714) 675-4070

RIGATONI - SPECIAL REQUEST
with yellow squash, sweet red peppers, onions and mushrooms in a hearty tomato sauce, topped with a dollop of fresh ricotta cheese. <u>*Request less oil (½ oz).*</u>
✓ CALORIES: Low (516)　　　✓✓ CHOLESTEROL: Very Low (25 mg)
✓ FAT: Low* (18 g)　　　✓ SODIUM: Low (392 mg) **
Exchanges: ¼ Meat, 3½ Bread, 3¾ Veg, 3¼ Fat

ANGEL HAIR ALLA CHECCA - SPECIAL REQUEST
served with Roma tomatoes, basil, garlic and extra virgin olive oil. <u>*Request less oil (½ oz).*</u>
✓ CALORIES: Low (470)　　　✓✓ CHOLESTEROL: Very Low (40 mg)
✓ FAT: Low* (16 g)　　　✓✓ SODIUM: Very Low (79 mg) **
Exchanges: 3¾ Bread, 2¼ Veg, 2¾ Fat

ANGEL HAIR - SPECIAL REQUEST
with artichoke hearts, sundried tomatoes, black olives, capers, herbed olive oil, and Italian parsley. <u>*Request just a touch of oil (1 tsp).*</u>
✓ CALORIES: Low (589)　　　✓✓ CHOLESTEROL: Very Low (60 mg)
✓ FAT: Low* (20 g)　　　SODIUM: High (1180 mg)
Exchanges: 3¾ Bread, 3¼ Veg, 4¾ Fat

CIAO CALIFORNIA SHRIMP SALAD - SPECIAL REQUEST
A refreshing blend of sweet red peppers, celery, oranges, sweet onions and tender shrimp with a delightfully different citrus dressing. <u>*Request dressing on the side (not included in analysis).*</u>
✓✓ CALORIES: Very Low (198)　　　✓ CHOLESTEROL: Low (120 mg)
✓✓ FAT: Very Low* (10 g)　　　✓✓ SODIUM: Very Low (149 mg) **
Exchanges: 1 Meat (extra lean), 1¼ Veg, ¼ Fruit, 1¾ Fat

PIZZA MARGHARITA WITH FAT-FREE CHEESE (½ PIZZA) - SPECIAL REQUEST
Roma tomatoes, fresh basil, mozzarella and garlic. Analysis is for ½ gourmet pizza. <u>*Request fat-free cheese.*</u>
✓ CALORIES: Low (488)　　　✓✓ CHOLESTEROL: Very Low (1 mg)
✓✓ FAT: Very Low* (8 g)　　　SODIUM: Moderate (974 mg) **
Exchanges: 2½ Meat, 4 Bread, ¾ Veg, 1¼ Fat

GOURMET VEGGIE PIZZA WITH FAT-FREE CHEESE (½ PIZZA) - SPECIAL REQUEST
Baby artichoke hearts, Spanish olives, capers, fresh herbs and mozzarella. Analysis is for ½ gourmet pizza. <u>*Request fat-free cheese.*</u>
✓ CALORIES: Low (493)　　　✓✓ CHOLESTEROL: None (0 mg)
✓✓ FAT: Very Low* (9 g)　　　SODIUM: High (1618 mg)
Exchanges: 2½ Meat, 4 Bread, 1 Veg, 1 Fat

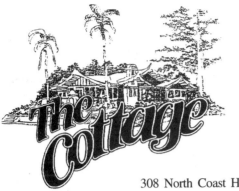

Welcome to The Cottage Restaurant, a landmark home that has watched the everchanging Laguna surf for more than a half century. We feature home-style cooking in an atmosphere that is seldom found in the modern-day stainless steel coffee shops or velvet-plush dinner houses. We hope you'll join the growing family of friends that make their dining out "home" The Cottage Restaurant. $$

The Cottage Restaurant
308 North Coast Hwy, Laguna Beach, CA 92651   (714) 494-3023

SHRIMP SCAMPI - SPECIAL REQUEST
sauteed in a basil-garlic butter and served with rice and vegetables.
Request less butter (½ oz) and vegetables steamed.
- ✓ CALORIES: Low (397)   CHOLESTEROL: Moderate (250 mg)
- ✓ FAT: Low (13 g)   ✓ SODIUM: Low (370 mg) **
  Exchanges: 2 Meat (extra lean), 2¼ Bread, ½ Veg, 2½ Fat

CIOPPINO - SPECIAL REQUEST
Scallops, jumbo shrimp, fresh fish, clams & herbs in a seafood tomato broth. Request less oil (½ oz).
- ✓✓ CALORIES: Very Low (331)   CHOLESTEROL: Moderate (221 mg)
- ✓ FAT: Low* (16 g)   SODIUM: Moderate (671 mg) **
  Exchanges: 3¾ Meat (extra lean), ¾ Veg, 2¾ Fat

SEAFOOD CATALINA - SPECIAL REQUEST
Sauteed sea scallops, jumbo shrimp, crab meat, Roma tomatoes, mushrooms, spinach and angel hair pasta tossed with olive oil. Request less oil (½ oz).
- ✓ CALORIES: Low (556)   CHOLESTEROL: Moderate (183 mg)
- ✓ FAT: Low* (17 g)   ✓ SODIUM: Low (462 mg) **
  Exchanges: 3¼ Meat (extra lean), 3¼ Bread, 1½ Veg, 2¾ Fat

BLACKENED SEA SCALLOPS - SPECIAL REQUEST
with roasted peppers, mushrooms, Roma tomatoes, garlic, herbs and olive oil, served with vegetables. Request less oil (½ oz) and vegetables steamed.
- ✓ CALORIES: Low (460)   ✓✓ CHOLESTEROL: Very Low (48 mg)
- ✓ FAT: Low* (18 g)   ✓ SODIUM: Low (409 mg) **
  Exchanges: 1¾ Meat (extra lean), 2¼ Bread, 1¾ Veg, 2¾ Fat

SHRIMP LOUISIANA
Spinach & fettuccine with sauteed prawns, cajun spices & green onions, served in a rich tomato broth.
- ✓ CALORIES: Low (545)   CHOLESTEROL: Moderate (262 mg)
- ✓ FAT: Low* (18 g)   SODIUM: Moderate (624 mg) **
  Exchanges: 2½ Meat (extra lean), 3¼ Bread, 1 Veg, 2¾ Fat

SANTA FE ANGEL HAIR PASTA - SPECIAL REQUEST
Spiced chicken strips, roasted peppers, mushrooms, sun dried tomatoes & olive oil with white wine sauce. Request less oil (½ oz).
- CALORIES: Moderate (687)   ✓ CHOLESTEROL: Low (130 mg)
- ✓ FAT: Low (15 g)   ✓✓ SODIUM: Very Low (229 mg) **
  Exchanges: 6¾ Meat (extra lean), 3¼ Bread, ½ Veg, 1¼ Fat

* Primarily unsaturated fat
** If you request no added salt

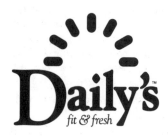

When cardiac surgeon Pat Daily couldn't find a quick-service restaurant that prepared good-tasting, low-fat food -- the way he likes to eat -- he opened his own! <u>All of Daily's Fit & Fresh menu items contain fewer than 10 grams of fat and/or less than 20% of the calories from fat.</u> Daily's uses the freshest, highest quality ingredients and publishes the nutritional content on all the menu items. The menu includes an array of salads, sandwiches, hot pasta, grilled fish, fruit smoothies, and even low-fat desserts. Below are 5 of the most popular menu items. $

Daily's *fit & fresh*

Laguna Niguel: Laguna Niguel Marketplace, 27000 Alicia Parkway   FAX 831-9733   ph 831-8792
Tustin: Larwin Square Tustin, 498 E. First Street   FAX 730-6844   ph 730-7034

3-BEAN & CORN CHILI (VEGETARIAN)
with brown rice, a dollop of yogurt, and green salad.
✓✓ CALORIES: Very Low (283)   ✓✓ CHOLESTEROL: None (0 mg)
✓✓ FAT: Very Low* (3½ g)   ✓ SODIUM: Low (350 mg)
Exchanges: 3 Bread, ¾ Veg, ½ Fat

BAJA FLAVORS PASTA SALAD
Penne pasta, vegetables, kidney and black beans in a spicy Baja dressing.
✓✓ CALORIES: Low (350)   ✓✓ CHOLESTEROL: None (0 mg)
✓✓ FAT: Very Low* (8 g)   ✓ SODIUM: Low (380 mg)
Exchanges: 3½ Bread, 1¼ Veg, 1¼ Fat

GARDEN VEGETABLE BURGER
Served on a whole grain honey bun.
✓ CALORIES: Low (390)   ✓✓ CHOLESTEROL: None (0 mg)
✓✓ FAT: Very Low* (7 g)   ✓ SODIUM: Low (440 mg)
Exchanges: 3 Bread, 3¼ Veg, 1 Fat

DAILY'S SPICY, GRILLED CHICKEN PIZZA
Grilled chicken & red onions, peppers, spicy tomato marinade with skim milk mozzarella cheese on our whole wheat pizza crust.
✓ CALORIES: Low (467)   ✓✓ CHOLESTEROL: Very Low (60 mg)
✓✓ FAT: Very Low (8½ g)   ✓ SODIUM: Low (445 mg)
Exchanges: 2½ Meat, 3 Bread, 2 Veg, ½ Milk

CAJUN CATFISH
with black beans, brown rice and green salad.
✓✓ CALORIES: Very Low (322)   ✓✓ CHOLESTEROL: Very Low (65 mg)
✓✓ FAT: Very Low* (6 g)   ✓ SODIUM: Low (380 mg)
Exchanges: 2¾ Meat, 2 Bread, ½ Veg

Nutrition information supplied by Daily's.

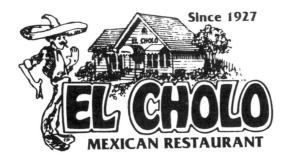

Since 1927

"A legend in its own time" according to Southern California Restaurant Writers. Over 65 years of superb cuisine at moderate prices. "The Mexican against which all others must be judged." - Zagat Survey. $

El Cholo Mexican Restaurant
840 Whittier Blvd.
La Habra, CA 90631   (714) 525-1320

SANTA FE VEGETARIAN TOSTADA

Verduras Asadas -- grilled vegetables (tomatoes, zucchini, chayote, green onions and fresh chiles) with a citrus vinaigrette and black beans with queso fresco. Avocado & fried tortilla not included in analysis.

✓ CALORIES: Low (352) ✓✓ CHOLESTEROL: Very Low (21 mg)
✓ FAT: Low (20 g) ✓ SODIUM: Low (332 mg) **
Exchanges: ½ Meat, 1 Bread, 2 Veg, ¼ Fruit, 3¼ Fat

PUERTO PENASCO SEAFOOD SALAD

Chilled shrimp, scallops, crabmeat and calamari in a lime-orange vinaigrette. Avocado and chips not included in analysis.

✓ CALORIES: Low (388) CHOLESTEROL: Moderate (212 mg)
✓ FAT: Low (20 g) SODIUM: Moderate (632 mg) **
Exchanges: 3½ Meat (extra lean), 1¼ Veg, ¼ Fruit, 3 Fat

EL CHOLO VEGETARIAN PLATTER

A rich spinach, mushroom and cheese enchilada, vegetable tamale, grilled vegetables, and vegetable taco with a pilonsillo eggplant puree.

CALORIES: Moderate (807) ✓✓ CHOLESTEROL: Very Low (20 mg)
✓ FAT: Low (18 g) ✓ SODIUM: Low (530 mg) **
Exchanges: ¾ Meat, 8¼ Bread, 1¼ Veg, ¼ Fruit, 2½ Fat

VEGETARIAN TACOS

Julienne of Mexican vegetables and plantain wrapped in a whole wheat tortilla with a honey-ancho chile sauce and served with rice & beans.

✓ CALORIES: Low (546) ✓✓ CHOLESTEROL: Very Low (8 mg)
✓ FAT: Low* (16 g) SODIUM: Moderate (847 mg) **
Exchanges: 3¾ Bread, ½ Veg, 1 Fruit, 3 Fat

---

* Primarily unsaturated fat
** If you request no added salt

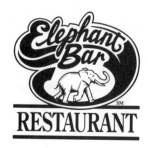

Unbelievable atmosphere, tropical, fun and casual with a great patio. Spectacular appetizers, elephant-size salads, super sandwiches and the best burgers in town. Favorites like sizzling Fajitas, Stir Fried Sesame Chicken, Charbroiled Tri-Tip, and Caribbean Pot Roast are big sellers. Stomp on down with friends to the Elephant Bar. It's always an adventure! $

Elephant Bar

14303 Firestone Blvd, La Mirada, CA 90638 (714) 994-1474
25250 East La Paz Road, Laguna Hills, CA 92653 (714) 470-0711

VEGETABLE TACOS WITH GRILLED CHICKEN
Soft warm corn tortillas filled with shredded lettuce, diced tomatoes, ranch beans, roasted peppers, onions and zucchini, topped with grilled chicken strips. Served with salsa & side of garden salad with non-fat dressing.

✓✓ CALORIES: Very Low (328) ✓✓ CHOLESTEROL: Very Low (39 mg)
✓✓ FAT: Very Low (4 g) ✓✓ SODIUM: Very Low (293 mg)

SIZZLING CHICKEN FAJITAS
Marinated skinless chicken breast charbroiled over peppers and onions. Served with ranch beans, salsa, shredded lettuce & warm corn tortillas.

CALORIES: Moderate (712) ✓ CHOLESTEROL: Low (105 mg)
✓✓ FAT: Very Low (8 g) SODIUM: High (2299 mg)

MEDITERRANEAN VEGETABLE PASTA
Penne pasta with artichoke hearts, diced tomatoes, garlic, mushrooms, sweet peppers, and Greek olives with tomato basil sauce and feta cheese.

CALORIES: Moderate (957) ✓✓ CHOLESTEROL: Very Low (28 mg)
✓ FAT: Low (14 g) SODIUM: High (1617 mg)

COBB SALAD SANDWICH
Whole wheat pita bread filled with chopped mixed greens, diced chicken breast, tomatoes, feta cheese, black olives, bean sprouts and chopped eggs, with non-fat Italian dressing. Served with low-fat penne pasta salad (not included in analysis).

CALORIES: Moderate (742) ✓✓ CHOLESTEROL: Very Low (33 mg)
✓✓ FAT: Very Low (8 g) SODIUM: High (2194 mg)

GUILTLESS CHOCOLATE PEANUT BUTTER YOGURT PIE†
Swirls of frozen non-fat chocolate and peanut butter yogurt with chunks of Reeses peanut butter cups.

CALORIES: Moderate (378) ✓✓ CHOLESTEROL: Very Low (5 mg)
✓ FAT: Low (5 g) SODIUM: Moderate (255 mg)

Nutrition information supplied by Elephant Bar.

† Side dish guidelines are 1/3 of entree guidelines

✓ Low ✓✓ Very Low

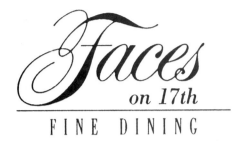

You'll find gourmet California Cuisine at the celebrity-themed Faces on 17th. This elegant-yet-comfortable restaurant features fresh fish, poultry and pasta from award-winning Chef Ali. Light, flavorful sauces provide healthy dining choices, with complete dinners offering true dining value. Your special requests are always welcome. Serving lunch Monday-Friday, dinner Monday-Saturday. Entertainment nightly in our candlelit lounge. $$

Faces on 17th

1615 East 17th Street, Santa Ana, CA 92705   (714) 972-2200

GRILLED SWORDFISH WITH MANDARIN ORANGE GINGER SAUCE
with potatoes, rice and vegetables.

✓ CALORIES: Low (422)   ✓ CHOLESTEROL: Low (88 mg)
✓ FAT: Low* (14 g)   ✓✓ SODIUM: Very Low (235 mg) **
Exchanges: 4½ Meat, 1½ Bread, ½ Veg, 1¼ Fat

FRESH FILET OF SALMON FLORENTINE - SPECIAL REQUEST
on a bed of sautéed spinach with a white wine & dill sauce, potatoes, rice and vegetables.
Request salmon poached & sauce on the side (sauce not included in analysis).

✓ CALORIES: Low (475)   ✓ CHOLESTEROL: Low (114 mg)
✓ FAT: Low* (20 g)   ✓✓ SODIUM: Very Low (296 mg) **
Exchanges: 5 Meat, 1½ Bread, 1 Veg, 1½ Fat

CHICKEN CALABRESE
Fresh charbroiled chicken breast, eggplant, bell pepper, tomato and onions, served with potatoes, rice and vegetables.

✓ CALORIES: Low (550)   CHOLESTEROL: Moderate (159 mg)
✓ FAT: Low (17 g)   ✓✓ SODIUM: Very Low (189 mg) **
Exchanges: 8 Meat (extra lean), 2 Bread, 1½ Veg, 2 Fat

SEAFOOD FETTUCCINE
Shrimp, scallops, and selected fresh fish in a light tomato-basil sauce.

✓ CALORIES: Low (557)   CHOLESTEROL: Moderate (182 mg)
✓ FAT: Low* (20 g)   ✓✓ SODIUM: Very Low (268 mg) **
Exchanges: 2¼ Meat (extra lean), 3½ Bread, ½ Veg, 3½ Fat

ANGEL HAIR CHECCA - SPECIAL REQUEST
Fresh tomato, sun-dried tomato and basil, sautéed in olive oil with Ricotta cheese. Request less oil (½ oz).

✓ CALORIES: Low (507)   ✓ CHOLESTEROL: Low (116 mg)
✓ FAT: Low* (20 g)   ✓✓ SODIUM: Very Low (183 mg) **
Exchanges: 4¼ Bread, ½ Veg, 3¾ Fat

---

* Primarily unsaturated fat
** If you request no added salt

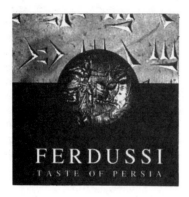

Persian cuisine is one of the unexpected. While its basic ingredients are familiar to most (such as lamb and rice), the ingredients that enhance it, while not unknown, are used infrequently in Western cuisine: pomegranates, pistachio nuts, saffron, dried lime, rosewater, yogurt, cardamon, cloves, barberry, fenugreek, the unique spice sumak -- the list is endless. Famous Lunch Buffet every Monday and Friday. Come enjoy... $$

The Taste of Persia
Ferdussi   (714) 545-9096
3605 S. Bristol Street, Santa Ana, CA 92704
at MacArthur Blvd, one block north of South Coast Plaza

APPETIZER: KASHK BODEMJON (EGGPLANT SPREAD)†
A medley of eggplants, "Kashk" (a dried yogurt sauce), with sauteed garlic, mint & onion.
✓ CALORIES: Low (161)   ✓✓ CHOLESTEROL: Very Low (¼ mg)
✓✓ FAT: Very Low* (1 g)   SODIUM: High (714 mg)**
Exchanges: 5¾ Veg

CHICKEN SHISH KABOB
Thick chunks of chicken, marinated in saffron yogurt sauce, skewered with onion, bell pepper and tomato and cooked on open flame. Served with fluffy basmati rice (see analysis below).
✓ CALORIES: Low (428)   CHOLESTEROL: Moderate (173 mg)
✓ FAT: Low (12 g)   ✓✓ SODIUM: Very Low (257 mg) **
Exchanges: 9 Meat (extra lean), 2 Veg, 1 Fat

BABY SALMON
Fresh filet of baby salmon dipped in saffron sauce and cooked on open fire.
Served with fluffy basmati rice (see analysis below).
✓✓ CALORIES: Very Low (322)   ✓ CHOLESTEROL: Low (143 mg)
✓ FAT: Low* (15 g)   ✓✓ SODIUM: Very Low (200 mg) **
Exchanges: 5¾ Meat

WHITE FISH KABOB
Fresh filet of white fish dipped in saffron sauce and cooked on open flame.
Served with fluffy basmati rice (see analysis below).
✓✓ CALORIES: Very Low (317)   ✓ CHOLESTEROL: Low (112 mg)
✓✓ FAT: Very Low* (6 g)   ✓✓ SODIUM: Very Low (257 mg) **
Exchanges: 5¾ Meat (extra lean)

BASMATI RICE† *(4 oz serving)*
✓ CALORIES: Low (158)   ✓✓ CHOLESTEROL: None (0 mg)
✓✓ FAT: Very Low* (1 g)   ✓✓ SODIUM: Very Low (1 mg) **
Exchanges: 2 Bread, ¼ Fat

† Side dish guidelines are 1/3 of entree guidelines
✓ Low   ✓✓ Very Low

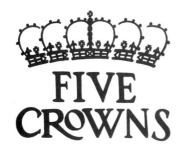

Five Crowns may be located in Corona del Mar, but its heart belongs to England. To this day the restaurant continues to be the most authentic reproduction of an English inn in North America. An award-winning menu of traditional favorites and seasonal specialties is served, including lobster tails, rack of lamb, fresh fish, pasta and chicken from the rotisserie. We take particular pride in our wines, having been chosen as a Wine Spectator Grand Award-winner since 1983, with over 800 labels at surprisingly reasonable prices.

$$

Five Crowns   3801 E. Coast Hwy, Corona del Mar, CA 92625   (714) 760-0331

PORCINI MUSHROOM RAVIOLI
Tossed with fresh tomatoes, basil, garlic and extra virgin olive oil.

✓ CALORIES: Low (372)   ✓✓ CHOLESTEROL: Very Low (50 mg)
✓ FAT: Low (14 g)   ✓ SODIUM: Low (456 mg) **
Exchanges: 5 Bread, 3 Veg, 1¼ Fat

GRILLED SALMON - SPECIAL REQUEST
Topped with a Portabello mushroom, tomato & mint salsa.
Request steamed vegetables and roasted red potatoes (included in analysis).

✓ CALORIES: Low (523)   ✓ CHOLESTEROL: Low (114 mg)
FAT: Moderate* (23 g)   ✓✓ SODIUM: Very Low (164 mg) **
Exchanges: 5 Meat, 1½ Bread, 2½ Veg, 1¾ Fat

BROILED NOVA SCOTIA LOBSTER TAILS - SPECIAL REQUEST
Three tails with fresh vegetables and lemon.
Request steamed vegetables and roasted red potatoes (included in analysis).

✓ CALORIES: Low (515)   CHOLESTEROL: Moderate (238 mg)
✓✓ FAT: Very Low (9 g)   SODIUM: High (1292 mg)
Exchanges: 5¾ Meat (extra lean), 1½ Bread, 2 Veg, 1¼ Fat

GRILLED SWORDFISH - SPECIAL REQUEST
with pineapple papaya salsa. Request steamed vegetables
and roasted red potatoes (included in analysis).

✓ CALORIES: Low (484)   ✓ CHOLESTEROL: Low (86 mg)
✓ FAT: Low* (16 g)   ✓✓ SODIUM: Very Low (257 mg) **
Exchanges: 4½ Meat, 1½ Bread, 2¼ Veg, ½ Fruit, 1½ Fat

STEAMED VEGETABLE PLATE - SPECIAL REQUEST
Request roasted potatoes. Sauce and Yorkshire pudding not included in analysis.

✓✓ CALORIES: Very Low (248)   ✓✓ CHOLESTEROL: Very Low (1 mg)
✓✓ FAT: Very Low (7 g)   ✓✓ SODIUM: Very Low (49 mg) **
Exchanges: 1½ Bread, 4¼ Veg, 1 Fat

---

* Primarily unsaturated fat
** If you request no added salt

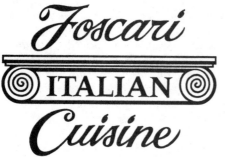

Foscari's Restaurant is the fulfillment of our family's long-cherished dream. Our love of fine Italian and Mediterranean cuisine has been enhanced by our travels throughout Europe. In business since 1975, we are eager to share our experience and culinary artistry with you. Foscari's is proud to offer you authentic recipes, fresh seafood, freshly made pasta & sauces, bread baked fresh daily, and pizzas from our wood-burning oven. $$

Foscari Italian Cuisine   (714) 779-1777
5645 East La Palma, Anaheim Hills, CA 92807

PENNE DEL SOLE
Penne pasta tossed with broccoli & sundried tomatoes in a light garlic sauce.
✓ CALORIES: Low (591)   ✓✓ CHOLESTEROL: None (0 mg)
✓ FAT: Low* (15 g)   ✓✓ SODIUM: Very Low (213 mg) **
Exchanges: 4¼ Bread, 1½ Veg, 2¾ Fat

RISOTTO AL CARCIOFFI - SPECIAL REQUEST
Arborio rice with artichoke hearts and pine nuts. <u>Request no oil or butter.</u>
✓ CALORIES: Low (527)   ✓✓ CHOLESTEROL: Very Low (1 mg)
✓ FAT: Low* (20 g)   ✓ SODIUM: Low (334 mg) **
Exchanges: 4¼ Bread, 2½ Veg, 4 Fat

RIGATONI AL POMODORO
Pasta tubes tossed in fresh tomato sauce with basil.
✓ CALORIES: Low (352)   ✓✓ CHOLESTEROL: None (0 mg)
✓✓ FAT: Very Low* (4 g)   SODIUM: High (1664 mg)
Exchanges: 3¾ Bread, 2 Veg, ½ Fat

LINGUINI ALLA VONGOLE & ARRABIATTA SAUCE
Thin pasta tossed with Manilla clams, garlic, olive oil and arrabiatta sauce.
✓ CALORIES: Low (546)   ✓✓ CHOLESTEROL: Very Low (39 mg)
✓ FAT: Low* (17 g)   SODIUM: High (1088 mg)
Exchanges: 2 Meat (extra lean), 3¾ Bread, 1¼ Veg, 3 Fat

GAMBERONI ALLA GRIGLIA
Jumbo fresh water prawns, olive oil and lemon, served with fresh vegetables.
✓ CALORIES: Low (405)   CHOLESTEROL: High (437 mg)
✓ FAT: Low* (18 g)   SODIUM: Moderate (901 mg) **
Exchanges: 4 Meat (extra lean), ¾ Veg, ½ Fruit, 2¾ Fat

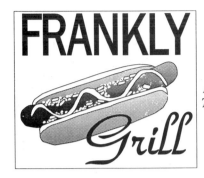

Wish you could eat sausage and hotdogs again?
Now at FRANKLY GRILL you CAN!
We're an upscale hotdog stand with a Healthy Twist.
Over ½ of our 12 varieties of gourmet Haute Links
are 100% lean chicken, turkey, or vegetarian base.
LOW-FAT, LOW-CALORIE & PRESERVATIVE-FREE!
Top with 7 gourmet mustards & vast array of toppings.
Really hungry?
Try a side of our homemade Low-fat Chili or Soup.
And there's always Micro Beers on Tap
to wash it all down! $

Frankly Grill   32371-D Golden Lantern, Laguna Niguel, CA 92677   (714) 248-7740
(next to Edward's Movie Theatre)

Help yourself to our 7 gourmet mustards and the following toppings which are all
fat-free and 35 calories or less per serving (not included in analysis below):
onions, tomatoes, sauerkraut, pickle relish, corn relish and diced peppers.

HOT TURKEY ITALIAN SAUSAGE SANDWICH

✓ CALORIES: Low (364)   ✓ CHOLESTEROL: Low (90 mg)
✓✓ FAT: Very Low (10 g)   SODIUM: Moderate (978 mg) **
Exchanges: 2¾ Meat, 2¾ Bread

CHICKEN APPLE SANDWICH OR EAST INDIAN SAUSAGE SANDWICH

✓ CALORIES: Low (378)   ✓ CHOLESTEROL: Low (89 mg)
✓ FAT: Low (13 g)   SODIUM: Moderate (969 mg) **
Exchanges: 2½ Meat, 3¼ Bread, 1¼ Fat

SWEET BASIL, TUSCANY, OR PICANTE CHICKEN SAUSAGE SANDWICH

✓ CALORIES: Low (402)   ✓ CHOLESTEROL: Low (101 mg)
✓ FAT: Low (16 g)   SODIUM: High (1078 mg) **
Exchanges: 2¾ Meat, 2¾ Bread, 1¼ Fat

VEGETARIAN HOT DOG

✓✓ CALORIES: Very Low (289)   ✓✓ CHOLESTEROL: None (0 mg)
✓✓ FAT: Very Low* (4 g)   SODIUM: Moderate (728 mg) **
Exchanges: 2¼ Meat (extra lean) 3 Bread

VEGETARIAN SANDWICH

✓ CALORIES: Low (358)   ✓✓ CHOLESTEROL: Very Low (30 mg)
✓ FAT: Low (12 g)   ✓ SODIUM: Low (549 mg) **
Exchanges: 1¼ Meat, 2¾ Bread, 1½ Veg, 1¼ Fat

GRILLED CHICKEN BREAST SANDWICH

✓ CALORIES: Low (370)   ✓ CHOLESTEROL: Low (87 mg)
✓✓ FAT: Very Low (6 g)   ✓ SODIUM: Low (501 mg) **
Exchanges: 5 Meat (extra lean), 2¾ Bread

SIDE DISH: HOMEMADE CHICKEN CHILI WITH BLACK BEANS *(6 oz cup)*
101 calories, 2 g fat, 18 mg cholesterol, 532 mg sodium**, Exch: ¾ Meat, ¾ Bread, ½ Veg

SIDE DISH: HOMEMADE ITALIAN GARDEN VEGETABLE SOUP *(6 oz cup)*
47 calories, ½ g fat*, 1 mg cholesterol, 538 mg sodium**, Exch: ½ Bread, ½ Veg

---

* Primarily unsaturated fat
** If you request no added salt   *Healthy Dining in Orange County*   **71**

GANDHI
INDIAN CUISINE

Gandhi is a breathtaking cultural experience -- a Gold Award-winning Indian restaurant in Southern California with an elegant decor and exceptional cuisine. Using only the freshest ingredients, Gandhi serves a variety of specialized Indian dishes which are prepared hot or mild depending on your preference. Lunch buffet, including many Healthy Dining selections, 11:30 am to 2:30 pm seven days a week. Dinner 5:30 to 10:00 pm Sunday thru Thursday and 5:30 to 11 pm Friday and Saturday. $$

Gandhi Indian Cuisine 1621-D Sunflower Ave., Santa Ana, CA 92704   556-7273

MUSHROOM BHAJEE
Fresh sauteed mushrooms.

✓✓ CALORIES: Very Low (157)   ✓✓ CHOLESTEROL: None (0 mg)
✓✓ FAT: Low* (7 g)   SODIUM: High (1121 mg) #
Exchanges: 2½ Veg, 1 Fat

BAINGAN MASALA
Fresh eggplant medallions cooked in masala curry.

✓✓ CALORIES: Very Low (200)   ✓✓ CHOLESTEROL: None (0 mg)
✓✓ FAT: Very Low* (9 g)   SODIUM: High (1118 mg) #
Exchanges: 1¼ Veg, ¾ Bread, 1½ Fat

CHICKEN TIKKA - SPECIAL REQUEST
Choice tender pieces of marinated spring chicken cooked in the tandoor with herbs and spices. Request white meat only.

✓ CALORIES: Low (471)   CHOLESTEROL: Moderate (173 mg)
✓ FAT: Low (16 g)   SODIUM: High (1262 mg) #
Exchanges: 9 Meat (extra lean), ¾ Veg, 1½ Fat

FISH TIKKA
Fresh fish of the day grilled in the tandoor and served in a curry sauce. Analysis is for swordfish; other fish similar.

✓ CALORIES: Low (381)   ✓ CHOLESTEROL: Low (89 mg)
✓ FAT: Low* (17 g)   SODIUM: High (1311 mg) #
Exchanges: 5 Meat (extra lean), ¼ Veg, 1½ Fat

VEGETABLE JALFREZI

✓✓ CALORIES: Very Low (214)   ✓✓ CHOLESTEROL: None (0 mg)
✓✓ FAT: Very Low* (8 g)   SODIUM: High (1146 mg) #
Exchanges: ¾ Bread, 2¾ Veg, 1½ Fat

RICE † (6 oz)
CALORIES: Moderate (233)   ✓✓ CHOLESTEROL: Very Low (3 mg)
✓✓ FAT: Very Low (2 g)   ✓✓ SODIUM: Very Low (2 mg)
Exchanges: 3¼ Bread, ¼ Fat

† Side dish guidelines are 1/3 of entree guidelines
# Sodium can be reduced on special request

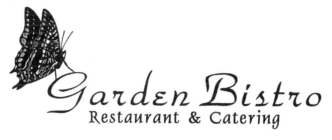

Garden Bistro
Restaurant & Catering

Step into the charming and colorful Mediterranean garden setting of Garden Bistro, where you will be hosted by award-winning chef Jim Parvin and treated to a mix of culinary delights from Italian to Mediterranean and contemporary Spa Cuisine. Among his creations are soups, salads, pasta and delicious desserts. Highly recommended for the sophisticated yet budget-minded. Open 11 am - 10 pm Mon-Sat, 11 am - 7 pm Sunday. $

Garden Bistro   Crystal Court, 2nd floor, South Coast Plaza   (714) 546-6004
3333 Bear Street, Costa Mesa, CA 92626

PENNE ARRABIATO
with sundried tomato, sauteed breast of chicken and rosemary.
✓ CALORIES: Low (599)   ✓✓ CHOLESTEROL: Very Low (65 mg)
✓ FAT: Low (12 g)   SODIUM: High (1378 mg)
Exchanges: 3½ Meat (extra lean), 2½ Bread, ¼ Veg, 1 Fat

PAPAYA & SPICED GRILLED SHRIMP SALAD
✓✓ CALORIES: Very Low (259)   CHOLESTEROL: Moderate (153 mg)
✓✓ FAT: Very Low* (4 g)   ✓✓ SODIUM: Very Low (259 mg) **
Exchanges: 1½ Meat (extra lean), 1 Veg, 2 Fruit, ½ Fat

SAUTEED BARBERRIES & CURRANTS IN SAFFRON RICE
& MARINATED BREAST OF CHICKEN
✓ CALORIES: Low (599)   ✓ CHOLESTEROL: Low (87 mg)
✓✓ FAT: Very Low (9 g)   ✓✓ SODIUM: Very Low (83 mg) **
Exchanges: 4½ Meat (extra lean), 4¼ Bread, 1 Fruit, 1 Fat

PAPILLON SALAD WITH SUNDRIED CRANBERRY, BASMATI RICE
AND BREAST OF CHICKEN *with a Dijon vinaigrette dressing*
✓ CALORIES: Low (553)   ✓✓ CHOLESTEROL: Very Low (65 mg)
✓ FAT: Low (12 g)   ✓✓ SODIUM: Very Low (141 mg) **
Exchanges: 3½ Meat (extra lean), 2¼ Bread, 1½ Veg, 2¾ Fruit, 1½ Fat

ANGEL HAIR
with steamed broccoli in spicy basil marinara sauce.
✓ CALORIES: Low (393)   ✓✓ CHOLESTEROL: None (0 mg)
✓✓ FAT: Very Low* (4 g)   SODIUM: Moderate (640 mg) **
Exchanges: 3 Bread, 3½ Veg

SEASONED CHICKEN KABOB WITH SAFFRON RICE
✓ CALORIES: Low (599)   ✓ CHOLESTEROL: Low (130 mg)
✓✓ FAT: Very Low (7 g)   ✓✓ SODIUM: Very Low (125 mg) **
Exchanges: 6¾ Meat (extra lean), 4¼ Bread, 1¾ Veg, ¼ Fat

* Primarily unsaturated fat
** If you request no added salt

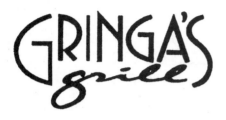

Have a taste for inventive Mexican cuisine with a California flair? Consider the healthy contemporary fare of Gringa's Grill on the Balboa Peninsula. Gringa's Grill is where "the locals go Latin" to enjoy exotic treats as well as traditional Mexican favorites. Everything is made from scratch -- we use nothing from a can. Accommodations for parties up to 60, catering, and full bar. Open for Sunday brunch and dinner daily. $

Gringa's Grill   111 Palm St., Balboa, CA 92661   (714) 723-6144

CHICKEN SOFT TACO
A corn tortilla filled with chopped cabbage, cotija cheese, green onions and chicken. Served with rice and calico beans (see analyses below).
✓✓ CALORIES: Very Low (178)   ✓✓ CHOLESTEROL: Very Low (37 mg)
✓✓ FAT: Very Low (7 g)   ✓✓ SODIUM: Very Low (292 mg) **
Exchanges: 1¾ Meat (extra lean), ¾ Bread, ¼ Veg, ¾ Fat

TWO GRILLED SHRIMP TACOS
Two of our famous grilled rock shrimp tacos. Served with rice & calico beans (analyses below).
✓ CALORIES: Low (409)   ✓ CHOLESTEROL: Low (120 mg)
✓ FAT: Low (16 g)   ✓ SODIUM: Low (540 mg) **
Exchanges: 1 Meat (extra lean), 2½ Bread, ½ Veg, 3 Fat

GRILLED FISH TACO
A flour tortilla filled with chopped cabbage, salsa blanco, green onions and grilled fish. Served with rice and calico beans (analyses below).
✓✓ CALORIES: Very Low (262)   ✓✓ CHOLESTEROL: Very Low (31 mg)
✓✓ FAT: Very Low (9 g)   ✓✓ SODIUM: Very Low (249 mg) **
Exchanges: 1¼ Meat (extra lean), 1¼ Bread, ½ Veg, 1½ Fat

GRILLED VEGETABLE SOFT TACO
A flour tortilla filled with chopped cabbage, green onions, cilantro and grilled vegetables. Served with rice and calico beans (analyses below).
✓✓ CALORIES: Very Low (150)   ✓✓ CHOLESTEROL: None (0 mg)
✓✓ FAT: Very Low (3 g)   ✓✓ SODIUM: Very Low (187 mg) **
Exchanges: 1¼ Bread, ¾ Veg, ½ Fat

MEDIA 4 MEDIA
Our home made beans and rice side by side in a bowl topped with cotija cheese and salsa.
CALORIES: Moderate (640)   ✓✓ CHOLESTEROL: Very Low (2 mg)
✓✓ FAT: Very Low* (4 g)   SODIUM: High (2283 mg)
Exchanges: 2¾ Meat, 7½ Bread, ¾ Veg, ¼ Fat

CALICO BEANS† *(5½ oz serving)*
CALORIES: Moderate (325)   ✓✓ CHOLESTEROL: None (0 mg)
✓✓ FAT: Very Low* (1 g)   SODIUM: Moderate (367 mg) **
Exchanges: 1¾ Meat, 3¾ Bread

RICE† *(3 oz)*
✓✓ CALORIES: Very Low (80)   ✓✓ CHOLESTEROL: Very Low (<1 mg)
✓✓ FAT: Very Low (<1 g)   SODIUM: High (775 mg)
Exchanges: 1 Bread, ¼ Veg

† Side dish guidelines are 1/3 of entree guidelines

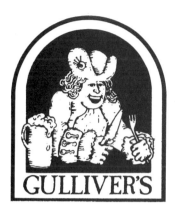

Gulliver's, famous for 24 years for its prime ribs of beef, also offers a number of low-fat, low-cholesterol, unique and tasty dishes. In the tradition of an old English tavern, you will be greeted and served by staff in authentic costume. Plenty of self-parking. Dress is casual. Lunch Mon-Fri 11:30am - 3pm; Dinner every night. Reservations suggested. $$

Gulliver's
18482 MacArthur Blvd.
Irvine, CA 92715   (714) 833-8411

GAZPACHO†
✓ CALORIES: Low (130)   ✓✓ CHOLESTEROL: None (0 mg)
   FAT: Moderate* (8 g)   SODIUM: High (972 mg)
Exchanges: 2½ Veg, 1½ Fat

FRESH KING SALMON - SPECIAL REQUEST
Request salmon poached and sauce on the side (sauce not included in analysis).
✓ CALORIES: Low (355)   ✓ CHOLESTEROL: Low (121 mg)
✓ FAT: Low* (14 g)   ✓✓ SODIUM: Very Low (293 mg) **
Exchanges: 5¾ Meat

ALASKAN HALIBUT - SPECIAL REQUEST
with mustard sauce and vegetable medley. *Request vegetables steamed*. Baked potato not included in analysis.
✓✓ CALORIES: Very Low (339)   ✓ CHOLESTEROL: Low (90 mg)
 ✓ FAT: Low* (11 g)   ✓ SODIUM: Low (538 mg) **
Exchanges: 4½ Meat (extra lean), ¾ Veg, ¼ Milk, 1 Fat

BREAST OF CHICKEN WITH MUSTARD SAUCE - SPECIAL REQUEST
Request steamed vegetables instead of souffle. Baked potato not included in analysis.
✓ CALORIES: Low (521)   CHOLESTEROL: Moderate (173 mg)
✓ FAT: Low (19 g)   ✓ SODIUM: Low (600 mg) **
Exchanges: 9 Meat (extra lean), 2 Veg, 2 Fat

WEST AUSTRALIAN LOBSTER TAIL - SPECIAL REQUEST
Request steamed vegetables instead of souffle. Butter & baked potato not included in analysis.
✓✓ CALORIES: Very Low (198)   ✓ CHOLESTEROL: Low (112 mg)
✓✓ FAT: Very Low* (5 g)   SODIUM: Moderate (667 mg) **
Exchanges: 3½ Meat (extra lean), ¾ Veg, ¾ Fat

---

* Primarily unsaturated fat
** If you request no added salt

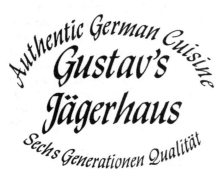

Authentic German Cuisine

Gustav's Jägerhaus

Sechs Generationen Qualität

Six generations ago, the Riker family opened its first Jägerhaus in Germany, serving juicy wild game dinners as the house specialty. Today, chef/owner Gus Riker still offers a wide variety of authentic German food, as well as great-tasting cook-it-yourself "rock" cuisine, which you grill on a greaseless tabletop stone. All dishes are prepared from scratch without artificial ingredients. Our friendly servers look forward to your visit. $

Gustav's Jägerhaus
2525 E. Ball Road, Anaheim, CA 92806 (714) 520-9500

"ROCK" FISH (COD)
Cook it yourself on a greaseless tabletop stone. Served with a medley of fresh vegetables. Sauces not included in analysis.
- ✓✓ CALORIES: Very Low (233)
- ✓ CHOLESTEROL: Low (85 mg)
- ✓✓ FAT: Very Low* (2 g)
- ✓✓ SODIUM: Very Low (137 mg) **

Exchanges: 3 Meat (extra lean), ¼ Bread, 1¾ Veg

"ROCK" CHICKEN
Cook it yourself on a greaseless tabletop stove. Served with a medley of fresh vegetables. Sauces not included in analysis.
- ✓ CALORIES: Low (366)
- CHOLESTEROL: Moderate (152 mg)
- ✓✓ FAT: Very Low (7 g)
- ✓✓ SODIUM: Very Low (147 mg) **

Exchanges: 8 Meat (extra lean), ¼ Bread, 1¾ Veg

"ROCK" VEGETABLES
A medley of fresh vegetables you cook yourself on a greaseless tabletop stone. Sauces not included in analysis.
- ✓✓ CALORIES: Very Low (99)
- ✓✓ CHOLESTEROL: None (0 mg)
- ✓✓ FAT: Very Low* (<1 g)
- ✓✓ SODIUM: Very Low (18 mg) **

Exchanges: ¾ Bread, 2 Veg

CHAR-BROILED CHICKEN BREAST SANDWICH
- ✓ CALORIES: Low (543)
- ✓ CHOLESTEROL: Low (111 mg)
- ✓ FAT: Low (12 g)
- SODIUM: Moderate (768 mg) **

Exchanges: 5½ Meat (extra lean), 3¾ Bread, ¼ Veg, 1¼ Fat

RECOMMENDED SIDE DISHES:
Green Beans (request steamed), Fruit Salad, Mashed Potatoes, Corn on the Cob

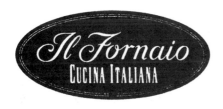

Enter Il Fornaio Cucina Italiana and feel as if you've been transported to Italy! Authentic Italian cuisine is served in a traditional trattoria-style setting. Munch on a basket of freshly baked breads and rolls while selecting from an extensive menu. Choose from a variety of homemade pastas, grilled meats and fowl from the rotisserie, pizzas from the wood-burning oven, and garden fresh salads. Be sure to save room for classic Italian desserts and espresso drinks. All major credit cards accepted. $$

Il Fornaio Cucina Italiana

18051 Von Karman Avenue, Irvine, CA 92715 (714) 261-1444

MANICHE AL POLLO - SPECIAL REQUEST
Elbow pasta, chicken breast, fresh broccoli, sundried tomatoes & roasted garlic.
<u>Request no butter and parmesan cheese on the side</u> (not included in analysis).
- ✓ CALORIES: Low (467)
- ✓✓ CHOLESTEROL: Very Low (67 mg)
- ✓ FAT: Low (18 g)
- ✓ SODIUM: Low (186 mg) **

Exchanges: 3½ Meat (extra lean), 2½ Bread, ¾ Veg, 2¾ Fat

PIZZA VEGETARIANA WITHOUT CHEESE (½ PIZZA)
Artichokes, zucchini, fresh tomatoes, red onions, sweet peppers, tomato sauce.
<u>Request no cheese</u>. Analysis is for ½ pizza without cheese.
- ✓ CALORIES: Low (351)
- ✓✓ CHOLESTEROL: None (0 mg)
- ✓ FAT: Low* (11 g)
- SODIUM: Moderate (567 mg) **

Exchanges: 1¼ Meat, 2¼ Bread, 1½ Veg, 1½ Fat

FUSILLI AI VEGETALI
Corkscrew pasta, fresh vegetables and herbs (no butter or oil).
- ✓ CALORIES: Low (558)
- ✓✓ CHOLESTEROL: Very Low (4 mg)
- ✓✓ FAT: Very Low* (3 g)
- ✓ SODIUM: Low (325 mg) **

Exchanges: 5¾ Bread, 2¼ Veg

PIATTO DI VEGETALI AL FORNO
A selection of fresh seasonal vegetables and garlic roasted in the wood-burning oven.
Served with polenta (not included in analysis).
- ✓ CALORIES: Low (306)
- ✓✓ CHOLESTEROL: None (0 mg)
- ✓ FAT: Low* (14 g)
- ✓✓ SODIUM: Very Low (29 mg) **

Exchanges: 1 Bread, 3½ Veg, 2¾ Fat

CAPELLINI AL POMODORO NATURALE
Angel hair pasta, chopped fresh roma tomatoes, basil, garlic & olive oil.
- ✓ CALORIES: Low (556)
- ✓✓ CHOLESTEROL: None (0 mg)
- ✓ FAT: Low* (16 g)
- ✓✓ SODIUM: Very Low (15 mg) **

Exchanges: 5½ Bread, ¾ Veg, 2¾ Fat

* Primarily unsaturated fat
** If you request no added salt

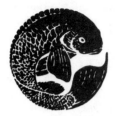

JOHN DOMINIS

John Dominis offers one of the most spectacular waterfront views in all of Southern California, a tropical atmosphere filled with lava rock pools, soothing waterfalls, and rich Koa wood furniture. More importantly, it features fine food, wonderful wines and great service. The menu includes a wide variety of contemporary Pacific seafood, beef, lamb and poultry selections, and a wine list consistently rated as one of the best by Wine Spectator Magazine. All these factors combine to make John Dominis a total dining experience and a special place to discover and enjoy on a regular basis. $$$

John Dominis
2901 West Coast Highway, Newport Beach, CA 92663   (714) 650-5112

BLACK AND BLUE SEARED TUNA
Hawaiian ahi blackened, then sliced and served with spicy Oriental noodles and orange sesame shoyu sauce and steamed vegetables.
✓ CALORIES: Low (453)   ✓✓ CHOLESTEROL: Very Low (74 mg)
✓ FAT: Low* (16 g)   SODIUM: High (2626 mg)
Exchanges: 3¼ Meat (extra lean), 1½ Bread, ¾ Veg, 2¾ Fat

GOLDEN CIOPPINO
An award-winning Dominis specialty. Oceans of shellfish simmered in an exotic Mediterranean broth with a slight hint of Pernod.
✓ CALORIES: Low (421)   ✓ CHOLESTEROL: Low (122 mg)
✓ FAT: Low* (18 g)   SODIUM: Moderate (831 mg) **
Exchanges: 3¼ Meat (extra lean), 4 Veg, 2¾ Fat

TIGER PRAWNS STIR-FRIED IN BLACK BEAN SAUCE
Large succulent prawns stir-fried in black beans, and served with steamed vegetables and rice (rice not included in analysis).
✓ CALORIES: Low (378)   CHOLESTEROL: High (440 mg)
✓✓ FAT: Very Low* (10 g)   SODIUM: High (2765 mg)
Exchanges: 4 Meat (extra lean), ¾ Bread, 1 Veg, 1½ Fat

GRILLED MAHI WITH SPICY YOGURT MANGO SAUCE - SPECIAL REQUEST
Mahi Mahi grilled with spicy mango sauce.
Request grilled and no nuts. Potato wafers not included in analysis.
✓✓ CALORIES: Very Low (320)   ✓ CHOLESTEROL: Low (126 mg)
✓✓ FAT: Very Low* (6 g)   ✓✓ SODIUM: Very Low (240 mg) **
Exchanges: 2¾ Meat (extra lean), ¼ Veg, 1¼ Fruit, ¾ Milk, 1 Fat

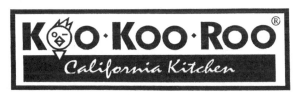

KOO KOO ROO California Kitchen features Original Skinless Flame-Broiled Chicken™, fresh oven-roasted turkey, rotisserie chicken, salads, and gourmet side dishes. Food is made fresh throughout the day and appeals to those who appreciate delicious, high quality, fresh food that can be enjoyed on the premises or as a home meal replacement. Catering available. $

Koo Koo Roo

Costa Mesa: 212 E. 17th St, Costa Mesa, CA 92627 (714) 631-1800
Irvine: 2963-A Michelson Drive, Irvine, CA 92715 Opening in 1996
Future 1996 locations: Tustin Market Place, Yorba Linda, 17th & Tustin, Aliso Viejo, Laguna Hills, San Clemente, Rancho Santa Margarita

---

ORIGINAL SKINLESS FLAME BROILED CHICKEN™ (¼ CHICKEN)
Includes breast and wing. Analyses for side dishes shown below.
- ✓ CALORIES: Low (394) CHOLESTEROL: Moderate (164 mg)
- ✓ FAT: Low (14 g) ✓ SODIUM: Low (580 mg)

Exchanges: 8½ Meat (extra lean), ¼ Veg, ¾ Fat

ORIGINAL SKINLESS FLAME BROILED CHICKEN™ (2 BREASTS)
Analyses for side dishes shown below.
- ✓ CALORIES: Low (503) CHOLESTEROL: Moderate (231 mg)
- ✓ FAT: Low (14 g) SODIUM: Moderate (628 mg)

Exchanges: 12 Meat (extra lean), ¼ Veg, ¾ Fat

ORIGINAL CHICKEN BREAST SANDWICH - SPECIAL REQUEST
Request no sandwich spread.
- ✓ CALORIES: Low (534) ✓ CHOLESTEROL: Low (116 mg)
- ✓✓ FAT: Very Low (9 g) SODIUM: Moderate (939 mg)

Exchanges: 6 Meat (extra lean), 3½ Bread, ¼ Veg, ½ Fat

TURKEY BREAST SANDWICH - SPECIAL REQUEST
Request no mayonnaise.
- ✓ CALORIES: Low (521) ✓ CHOLESTEROL: Low (118 mg)
- ✓✓ FAT: Very Low (7 g) SODIUM: Moderate (907 mg)

Exchanges: 6 Meat (extra lean), 3¼ Bread, ¼ Veg, 1 Fat

SIDE DISHES:

STEAMED VEGETABLES *(3¾ oz)* 34 calories, <1 g fat*, 0 cholesterol, 32 mg sodium; Exch: 1¼ Veg

BUTTERNUT SQUASH *(5½ oz)* 62 calories, < 1 g fat*, 0 cholesterol, 6 mg sodium; Exch: 1 Bread

TEN VEGETABLE SOUP# *(8¾ oz)* 88 calories, 2 g fat*, 0 cholesterol, 81 mg sodium

BAKED YAM# *(½ large)* 93 calories, <1 g fat, 0 cholesterol, 9 mg sodium

#Nutrition information for soup and yam supplied by Koo Koo Roo

* Primarily unsaturated fat
** If you request no added salt

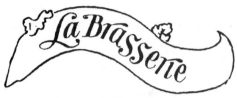

French Restaurant

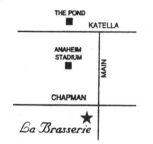

THE POND
KATELLA

ANAHEIM
STADIUM

MAIN

CHAPMAN

★
La Brasserie

La Brasserie is a warm, comfortable, easy-going French Restaurant in the Country Style, with an outstanding wine and champagne presentation. We have had nothing but kind words from the restaurant critics and have won many awards. Lunch is served Monday through Friday, dinner Monday through Saturday. We invite groups up to 60 people to use our new banquet room and can tailor a menu to meet your requests. Host Paul Rossi would like you to visit La Brasserie Restaurant, and Chef Joseph Vieillemaringe would love to cook for you. $$$

La Brasserie French Restaurant

202 South Main Street
Orange, CA 92668   (714) 978-6161

BROILED FILET OF SOLE - SPECIAL REQUEST
with steamed vegetables. <u>*Request no butter or oil & sauce on the side*</u>
(not included in analysis).

✓✓ CALORIES: Very Low (302)   ✓ CHOLESTEROL: Low (130 mg)
✓✓ FAT: Very Low (7 g)   ✓✓ SODIUM: Very Low (244 mg) **
Exchanges: 3¾ Meat (extra lean), ½ Bread, 1¼ Veg, ¾ Fat

SCAMPI PROVENCALE - SPECIAL REQUEST
with steamed vegetables. <u>*Request less oil (1 Tbs)*</u>.

✓ CALORIES: Low (372)   CHOLESTEROL: (306 mg)
✓ FAT: Low* (16 g)   ✓ SODIUM: Low (373 mg) **
Exchanges: 2¾ Meat (extra lean), ½ Bread, 2 Veg, 2¾ Fat

BROILED VEAL BELLE VERONIQUE - SPECIAL REQUEST
with steamed vegetables. <u>*Request no butter or oil & sauce on the side*</u>
(not included in analysis).

✓ CALORIES: Low (388)   ✓ CHOLESTEROL: Low (124 mg)
✓ FAT: Low (20 g)   ✓✓ SODIUM: Very Low (115 mg) **
Exchanges: 3¾ Meat, ½ Bread, 1¼ Veg, 2¾ Fat

BROILED ENGLISH DOVER SOLE - SPECIAL REQUEST
with steamed vegetables. <u>*Request no butter or oil & sauce on the side*</u>
(not included in analysis).

✓ CALORIES: Low (463)   CHOLESTEROL: Moderate (209 mg)
✓✓ FAT: Very Low* (9 g)   ✓ SODIUM: Low (344 mg) **
Exchanges: 6½ Meat (extra lean), ½ Bread, 1¼ Veg, 1 Fat

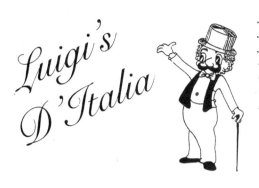

For over 15 years, Luigi's has been a favorite of the locals. You will enjoy the friendly, lively atmosphere created by this family owned and operated Italian restaurant. An extensive menu includes delicious chicken and baked specialties, pizza, sandwiches, salads, veal and seafood, a catch of the day, and Luigi's famous pasta specialties. $$

Luigi's D'Italia

801 S. State College Boulevard
Anaheim, CA 92806   (714) 490-0990

VEGETARIAN CHEESELESS PIZZA (2 SLICES) - SPECIAL REQUEST
with artichoke hearts, bell peppers, mushrooms, onions, tomatoes & eggplant.
Request eggplant grilled. Analysis is for 2 slices of a medium pizza.
- ✓ CALORIES: Low (527)
- ✓✓ CHOLESTEROL: None (0 mg)
- ✓ FAT: Low* (17 g)
- ✓ SODIUM: Low (572 mg) **

Exchanges: 4¼ Bread, 2¾ Veg, 3 Fat

LINGUINE AGLIO E OLIO
with garlic, olive oil and Italian seasonings.
- CALORIES: Moderate (616)
- ✓✓ CHOLESTEROL: None (0 mg)
- ✓ FAT: Low* (16 g)
- ✓✓ SODIUM: Very Low (23 mg) **

Exchanges: 5¾ Bread, 2¼ Veg, 2¾ Fat

HALIBUT LIVORNESE - SPECIAL REQUEST
prepared with oil, tomatoes, white wine and clam juice. Analysis is for halibut; other fish similar. Request less oil (¼ oz).
- ✓ CALORIES: Low (508)
- ✓ CHOLESTEROL: Low (91 mg)
- ✓ FAT: Low* (16 g)
- SODIUM: Moderate (715 mg) **

Exchanges: 5½ Meat (extra lean), 4¼ Veg, 1¾ Fat

NEW ZEALAND MUSSELS WITH RED SAUCE
over a large 11 oz serving of linguini with red sauce.
- CALORIES: Moderate (817)
- ✓✓ CHOLESTEROL: Very Low (63 mg)
- ✓ FAT: Low* (20 g)
- SODIUM: High (1367 mg)

Exchanges: 2 Meat (extra lean), 5¾ Bread, 6 Veg, 2¾ Fat

FETTUCCINE PRIMAVERA WITH TOMATO SAUCE
Tomato sauce, carrots, broccoli, zucchini, garlic and white wine.
- CALORIES: Moderate (730)
- ✓✓ CHOLESTEROL: None (0 mg)
- ✓ FAT: Low* (17 g)
- ✓ SODIUM: Low (351 mg) **

Exchanges: 5¾ Bread, 7 Veg, 2¾ Fat

* Primarily unsaturated fat
** If you request no added salt

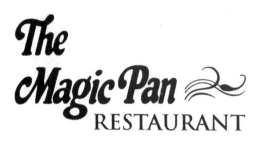

The Magic Pan has been a favorite eating establishment for over 25 years, featuring delicious crepes, fresh salads, homemade soups, original pasta dishes, and a wonderful selection of seafood, beef, and chicken dishes. Located in the South Coast Plaza Shopping Center, it is the perfect place to eat while shopping. Also, join us in the evening for dinner or one of our famous homemade strawberry crepe desserts. Our outside entrance allows us to serve nightly until 10 pm. $

The Magic Pan

South Coast Plaza, 3333 Bristol St., Costa Mesa, CA 92626   (714) 556-1225

ORANGE ALMOND SALAD - SPECIAL REQUEST
Our specialty. Romaine lettuce, toasted almonds and mandarin oranges with our famous sweet and sour dressing. Request dressing on the side (not included in analysis).
- ✓✓ CALORIES: Very Low (111)   ✓✓ CHOLESTEROL: None (0 mg)
- ✓✓ FAT: Very Low* (5 g)   ✓✓ SODIUM: Very Low (80 mg) **
- Exchanges: ½ Veg, ¼ Fruit, ¾ Fat

ORIENTAL CHICKEN SALAD
Romaine lettuce topped with teriyaki glazed chicken breast pieces, toasted almonds, water chestnuts, sesame seeds, mandarin orange slices & green onion. Dressing served on the side (not included in analysis).
- ✓ CALORIES: Low (400)   ✓ CHOLESTEROL: Low (87 mg)
- ✓ FAT: Low (16 g)   ✓ SODIUM: Low (385 mg) **
- Exchanges: 4½ Meat (extra lean), 2 Veg, ¼ Fruit, 1¾ Fat

LEMON LINGUINI WITH ARTICHOKES - SPECIAL REQUEST
Artichoke hearts, fresh tomatoes, capers and fresh basil sautéed in garlic and olive oil, tossed with a tangy lemon linguini. Request less oil (½ oz) and parmesan cheese on the side (cheese not included in analysis).
- ✓ CALORIES: Low (444)   ✓✓ CHOLESTEROL: None (0 mg)
- ✓ FAT: Low* (16 g)   ✓ SODIUM: Low (383 mg) **
- Exchanges: 3½ Bread, 2½ Veg, ¼ Fruit, 3 Fat

CAPELLINI WITH TOMATO AND FRESH BASIL - SPECIAL REQUEST
Fresh diced tomatoes, fresh basil, garlic and marinara sauce sautéed in olive oil and tossed with angel hair pasta. Request less oil (½ oz) and parmesan cheese on the side (cheese not included in analysis).
- ✓ CALORIES: Low (530)   ✓✓ CHOLESTEROL: None (0 mg)
- ✓ FAT: Low* (20 g)   ✓ SODIUM: Low (471 mg) **
- Exchanges: 4¾ Bread, ½ Veg, 3¼ Fat

CAPELLINI WITH SEAFOOD MARINARA - SPECIAL REQUEST
Baby clams, shrimp and scallops sautéed in olive oil with a fresh basil & garlic marinara sauce, served over a bed of angel hair pasta. Request less oil (½ oz).
- CALORIES: Moderate (617)   ✓ CHOLESTEROL: Low (109 mg)
- ✓ FAT: Low* (20 g)   ✓ SODIUM: Low (537 mg) **
- Exchanges: 2¼ Meat (extra lean), 4½ Bread, 3 Fat

Mandarin Taste Restaurant

川湘園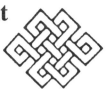

The elegant Mandarin Taste Restaurant features Hunan-Szechuan fare for everyone's palate, including an array of "Hot & Spicy" and "Slimmer's Choice" selections. The chefs take great pride with every dish -- with the freshest vegetables, meats, seafoods, and seasonings cooked with great care. Each selection is presented as a work of art, arranged and garnished to please the eye as well as the taste buds. We also invite you to try our all-you-can-eat Sunday Champagne Brunch or Happy Hour Monday-Friday, 4-7 pm. $$

Irvine: 14825 Jeffrey Rd., Irvine, CA 92720	(714) 651-8898
Diamond Bar: 23391 E. Golden Springs Dr., Diamond Bar, CA 91765	(909) 861-1819
Anaheim Hills: 5555 E. Santa Ana Canyon Rd., Anaheim Hills, CA 92807	(714) 974-8889
Lake Forest: 23600 Rockfield Blvd, Lake Forest, CA 92630	(714) 830-9984

CHINESE CHICKEN SALAD
✓✓ CALORIES: Very Low (281)   ✓✓ CHOLESTEROL: Very Low (43 mg)
✓ FAT: Low (20 g)   ✓✓ SODIUM: Very Low (194 mg) **
Exchanges: 2¼ Meat (extra lean), ¼ Bread, ½ Veg, 3½ Fat

HOMEBOUND NESTED - SPECIAL REQUEST
Shrimp and scallops stirred with snow peapods, bamboo shoots and mushrooms in a delicate nest which symbolizes home. Request steamed.
✓✓ CALORIES: Very Low (303)   CHOLESTEROL: Moderate (226 mg)
✓✓ FAT: Very Low* (4 g)   ✓ SODIUM: Low (373 mg) **
Exchanges: 4¼ Meat (extra lean), ¼ Bread, 1¾ Veg

SAUTEED SHRIMP
Marinated shrimp sauteed with special light sauce with a bit of Chinese wine.
✓✓ CALORIES: Very Low (223)   CHOLESTEROL: High (368 mg)
✓✓ FAT: Very Low* (4 g)   SODIUM: High (1386 mg)
Exchanges: 3¼ Meat (extra lean)

SLICED CHICKEN WITH MUSHROOMS AND PEA PODS - SPECIAL REQUEST. *Request steamed.*
✓✓ CALORIES: Very Low (346)   ✓ CHOLESTEROL: Low (130 mg)
✓✓ FAT: Very Low (6 g)   ✓✓ SODIUM: Very Low (204 mg) **
Exchanges: 6¾ Meat (extra lean), ½ Bread, 1 Veg

STEAMED WHOLE FISH (ROCK COD)
✓✓ CALORIES: Very Low (253)   ✓ CHOLESTEROL: Low (99 mg)
✓✓ FAT: Very Low* (2 g)   SODIUM: High (1813 mg)
Exchanges: 3½ Meat (extra lean), ¾ Veg

---

* Primarily unsaturated fat
** If you request no added salt

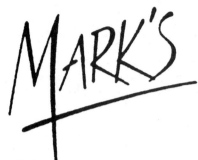

Nestled in the heart of downtown Laguna on Pacific Coast Highway, Mark's offers an atmosphere that hums with conversation, music and the sizzle of the finest in California cuisine. The atmosphere is casual, but "chic" -- definitely a place to experince. Open seven days a week, 5 pm - 10 pm; Sunday brunch 9 am - 3 pm. Call Mark's to inquire about their classical guitarist and reggae/calypso music performances. Reservations suggested. $$

Mark's   858 South Coast Highway, Laguna Beach, CA 92651   (714) 494-6711

CORN CHOWDER† - SPECIAL REQUEST
(10 oz) <u>Request no cream.</u>

✓ CALORIES: Low (153)   ✓✓ CHOLESTEROL: None (0 mg)
✓✓ FAT: Very Low* (1 g)   ✓✓ SODIUM: Very Low (13 mg) **
Exchanges: 2¼ Bread, ¼ Veg

BASIL-GARLIC RIGATONI - SPECIAL REQUEST
Chicken, fresh Roma tomatoes, sundried tomatoes, pine nuts, marjoram and sage. <u>*Request no butter.*</u>

✓ CALORIES: Low (533)   CHOLESTEROL: Moderate (161 mg)
✓ FAT: Low (12 g)   ✓✓ SODIUM: Very Low (128 mg) **
Exchanges: 3½ Meat (extra lean), 3 Bread, ½ Veg, 2 Fat

FIVE SPICED ALBACORE - SPECIAL REQUEST
Grilled and topped with five-spice ginger sauce and served with vegetables & rice. <u>*Request no oil and vegetables steamed.*</u>

✓ CALORIES: Low (481)   ✓ CHOLESTEROL: Low (101 mg)
✓ FAT: Low* (16 g)   SODIUM: High (2342 mg)
Exchanges: 6¼ Meat (extra lean), 1½ Bread, ¾ Veg, 2¼ Fat

MEDALLIONS OF TURKEY - SPECIAL REQUEST
Sautéed, with lemon, butter and capers, served with vegetables and garlic-mashed potatoes (mashed potatoes not included in analysis). <u>*Request no butter and vegetables steamed.*</u>

✓✓ CALORIES: Very Low (297)   ✓✓ CHOLESTEROL: Very Low (66 mg)
✓ FAT: Low (17 g)   ✓ SODIUM: Low (360 mg) **
Exchanges: 2¾ Meat (extra lean), ¾ Veg, 2¾ Fat

CHARBROILED VEGETABLE PIZZA (½ PIZZA)
Marinated charbroiled vegetables of the season and mozzarella cheese. Analysis is for ½ pizza.

✓ CALORIES: Low (437)   ✓✓ CHOLESTEROL: Very Low (16 mg)
✓ FAT: Low (20 g)   ✓ SODIUM: Low (549 mg) **
Exchanges: 1 Meat, 2¾ Bread, ¼ Veg, 3¼ Fat

† Side dish guidelines are 1/3 of entree guidelines

✓ Low   ✓✓ Very Low

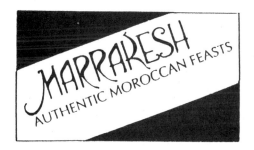

A splash of Morocco in Southern California, this exquisitely decorated restaurant is authentic from its inlaid tables to its superb gourmet Moroccan cuisine. Enjoy a fun and exotic feast in the Moroccan tradition featuring belly dancing. Open for dinner from 5 to 11 pm. Reservations suggested. $$

Marrakesh

1100 West Pacific Coast Hwy, Newport Beach, CA 92663   (714) 645-8384

SHRIMP BROCHETTE
Marinated jumbo shrimp grilled on skewers. Analyses for soup, salad, and rice below.
✓✓ CALORIES: Very Low (223)   CHOLESTEROL: Moderate (175 mg)
✓ FAT: Low* (13 g)   SODIUM: Moderate (670 mg) **
Exchanges: 1¾ Meat (extra lean), ¾ Veg, 2¼ Fat

CHICKEN BROCHETTE
Marinated pieces of chicken breast grilled on skewers. Analyses for soup, salad and rice below.
✓ CALORIES: Low (425)   CHOLESTEROL: Moderate (198 mg)
✓ FAT: Low (12 g)   ✓ SODIUM: Low (366 mg) **
Exchanges: 10¼ Meat (extra lean), ¾ Fat

FISH TAGINE
Fillet of fish marinated in fresh herbs and a hint of garlic, then baked with tomatoes and bell pepper. Served with harira soup and salad (analyses below).
✓ CALORIES: Low (438)   ✓✓ CHOLESTEROL: Very Low (73 mg)
✓ FAT: Low* (19 g)   ✓ SODIUM: Low (328 mg) **
Exchanges: 4½ Meat (extra lean), ½ Bread, 1¼ Veg, 2¾ Fat

VEGETABLE COUSCOUS
Steamed cracked wheat topped with fresh vegetables and raisins. Served with harira soup and salad (analyses below).
✓ CALORIES: Low (600)   ✓✓ CHOLESTEROL: None (0 mg)
✓✓ FAT: Very Low* (6 g)   ✓ SODIUM: Low (410 mg) **
Exchanges: 7 Bread, 2¼ Veg, ¼ Fruit, ¾ Fat

HARIRA LENTIL & GARBANZO SOUP
240 calories; 2 g fat*, 27 mg cholesterol, 935 mg sodium**, Exch: ½ Meat, 2½ Bread, 1¼ Veg, ¼ Fat

MOROCCAN RICE WITH PEAS, ALMONDS & RAISINS *(8 oz)*
296 calories, 6 g fat, 0 cholesterol, 439 mg sodium**, Exch: 3 Bread, ½ Fruit, 1 Fat

CUCUMBER AND TOMATO SALAD
84 calories, 6 g fat*, 0 cholesterol, 209 mg sodium**, Exch: ¾ Veg, 1 Fat

COOKED CARROT SALAD
87 calories, 1 g fat*, 0 cholesterol, 259 mg sodium**, Exch: 4 Veg

---

* Primarily unsaturated fat
** If you request no added salt

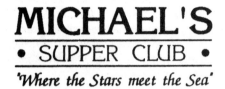

MICHAEL'S
• SUPPER CLUB •
'Where the Stars meet the Sea'

With an exquisite location on the island in Dana Point Harbor, Michael's offers spectacular waterfront dining and world-class cuisine from around the world. When you've finished, head upstairs and dance the night away at the only live entertainment dance club in the harbor. Dinner from 5:00 pm. Waterfront banquet facilities available, accommodating up to 250 guests. Live entertainment Wed - Sat at 9:00 pm. Happy Hour upstairs 3 pm - 7 pm. $$

Michael's Supper Club

24399 Dana Drive, Dana Point, CA 92629 (714) 240-7200

GREEK SALAD - SPECIAL REQUEST
Fresh crisp greens tossed with roma tomatoes, chopped bell peppers, Bermuda onions, cucumbers, calamata olives, Feta cheese and our Grecian herb dressing.
<u>Request dressing on the side</u> (not included in analysis).
✓✓ CALORIES: Very Low (139)   ✓✓ CHOLESTEROL: Very Low (25 mg)
✓✓ FAT: Very Low (8 g)   ✓ SODIUM: Low (460 mg) **
Exchanges: ½ Meat, 1¼ Veg, 1 Fat

PASTA PRIMAVERA WITH MARINARA SAUCE - SPECIAL REQUEST
Fresh garden vegetables seared in crushed garlic and extra virgin olive oil, served over a steaming bed of fettuccine. <u>Request marinara sauce and less oil (¼ oz)</u>.
✓ CALORIES: Low (415)   ✓✓ CHOLESTEROL: Very Low (62 mg)
✓ FAT: Low* (15 g)   ✓ SODIUM: Low (396 mg) **
Exchanges: ½ Meat, 2¾ Bread, 2¾ Veg, 2½ Fat

TARRAGON SCALLOPS FLORENTINE - SPECIAL REQUEST
Jumbo scallops rolled in tarragon and crushed pepper, simmered in a dry white wine and served on a bed of fresh steamed spinach with vegetables. <u>Request vegetables steamed</u>.
✓ CALORIES: Low (431)   ✓ CHOLESTEROL: Low (87 mg)
✓✓ FAT: Very Low (6 g)   SODIUM: Moderate (724 mg) **
Exchanges: 2¾ Meat, ¼ Bread, 2¾ Veg, 1¾ Milk, ¾ Fat

ROASTED EGGPLANT WITH SPINACH FETTUCCINE - SPECIAL REQUEST
Lightly seasoned thin-sliced eggplant, roasted and tossed with spinach fettuccine, fresh roma tomato sauce, garlic and Feta cheese. <u>Request less oil (¼ oz) and less cheese (½ oz)</u>.
✓ CALORIES: Low (517)   ✓✓ CHOLESTEROL: Very Low (12 mg)
✓ FAT: Low (20 g)   ✓✓ SODIUM: Very Low (282 mg) **
Exchanges: ¼ Meat, 3¾ Bread, 2½ Veg, 3½ Fat

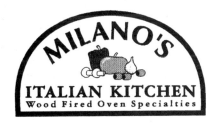

Milano's Italian Kitchen is a full service restaurant serving Northern Italian food with a California influence. Our dishes are generous enough to share and are made with the freshest ingredients. We serve salads, sandwiches, pastas, pizzas, rotisserie and grill specialities, as well as desserts, cappuccino and expresso.

$

Milano's Italian Kitchen

14210 Culver Drive, Irvine, CA   92714   (714) 857-8265

TUTTI COLORI PAPPARDELLE - SPECIAL REQUEST
with chicken, sun-dried tomatoes, peppers, mushrooms, roasted eggplant and garlic.
<u>*Request no butter or oil.*</u>

    CALORIES: Moderate (624)   ✓ CHOLESTEROL: Low (87 mg)
✓✓ FAT: Very Low (9 g)   ✓ SODIUM: Low (475 mg)**
    Exchanges: 4½ Meat (extra lean), 4½ Bread, 1¾ Veg, ¾ Fat

FETTUCCINE AL FRUTTI DI MARE - SPECIAL REQUEST
with shrimp, scallops, clams, roasted garlic & basil in a spicy tomato sauce. <u>*Request no oil.*</u>

   ✓ CALORIES: Low (533)   CHOLESTEROL: Moderate (173 mg)
✓✓ FAT: Very Low* (8 g)   ✓ SODIUM: Low (595 mg)**
    Exchanges: 3½ Meat (extra lean), 3¾ Bread, 1¾ Veg, 1¼ Fat

TAGLIATELLE DEL GIARDINO - SPECIAL REQUEST
Fettuccine with julienned seasonal vegetables tossed in a white wine and tomato-basil sauce. <u>*Request no butter or oil.*</u>

 ✓ CALORIES: Low (439)   ✓✓ CHOLESTEROL: None (0 mg)
✓✓ FAT: Very Low* (3 g)   ✓✓ SODIUM: Very Low (101 mg)**
    Exchanges: 4¼ Bread, 3¾ Veg, ¼ Fat

CAPPELLINI POMODORO - SPECIAL REQUEST
Fresh ripened tomatoes, garlic and fresh basil. <u>*Request no oil.*</u>

 ✓ CALORIES: Low (433)   ✓✓ CHOLESTEROL: None (0 mg)
✓✓ FAT: Very Low* (4 g)   ✓✓ SODIUM: Very Low (160 mg)**
    Exchanges: 4¼ Bread, 3¾ Veg, ¼ Fat

ORIENTAL LIME CHICKEN SALAD - SPECIAL REQUEST
with mixed greens, peanuts, sesame seeds and crispy noodles all tossed in a mustard vinaigrette. <u>*Request dressing and crispy noodles on the side*</u> *(not included in analysis).*

 ✓ CALORIES: Low (453)   ✓ CHOLESTEROL: Low (108 mg)
 ✓ FAT: Low (20 g)   ✓ SODIUM: Low (407 mg)**
    Exchanges: 5¾ Meat (extra lean), ¼ Veg, 3 Fat

* Primarily unsaturated fat
** If you request no added salt

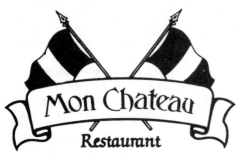

Mon Chateau
Restaurant
Belgian and French Cuisine

In the best tradition of French and Belgian cuisine, Mon Chateau places a strong emphasis on creating classical dishes with lighter sauces for today's discerning palate. Chef Timothy Plumb prepares tantalizing selections with the utmost care, select ingredients, and extreme pride... ENJOY! $$

Mon Chateau Restaurant
23642 El Toro Rd., Lake Forest, CA 92630
(714) 830-3810

SOUP DU JOUR - CARROT SOUP†
Soup changes daily. Other vegetable soups similar.
✓✓ CALORIES: Very Low (58)   ✓✓ CHOLESTEROL: Very Low (12 mg)
✓ FAT: Low (4 g)   SODIUM: High (606 mg)
Exchanges: ½ Veg, ¾ Fat

SAUMON FRAIS AUX HOMARD
Fresh, out-of-the-water poached salmon in lobster sauce laced with fine sherry and garnished with chives.
✓ CALORIES: Low (523)   ✓ CHOLESTEROL: Low (130 mg)
✓ FAT: Low (16 g)   SODIUM: Moderate (778 mg) **
Exchanges: 5¾ Meat, 1½ Bread, ¼ Milk, ¼ Fat

SCALLOPS FRAÎCHE MEUNIERE - SPECIAL REQUEST
Magnificent sea scallops sautéed with fresh lemon juice, parsley and chives.
Request less butter (¾ oz).
✓✓ CALORIES: Very Low (284)   ✓ CHOLESTEROL: Low (107 mg)
✓ FAT: Low (19 g)   ✓ SODIUM: Low (477 mg) **
Exchanges: 2¼ Meat (extra lean), 3½ Fat

POULET AUX FINES HERBES - SPECIAL REQUEST
A supreme, gratifying breast of chicken with fine herbs intensified by a white wine chicken velouté. Request less oil (¼ oz) and no butter.
✓ CALORIES: Low (421)   CHOLESTEROL: Moderate (173 mg)
✓ FAT: Low (14 g)   ✓✓ SODIUM: Very Low (225 mg) **
Exchanges: 9 Meat (extra lean), ¼ Bread, ¼ Veg, 1¼ Fat

CUISSE DE GRENOUILLE GASTON CLEMENT - SPECIAL REQUEST
Our one-of-a-kind house specialty! Lightly sautéed and garlicky frog legs deglazed with white wine and herbs. Request less oil (¼ oz) and less butter (½ oz).
✓ CALORIES: Low (363)   ✓ CHOLESTEROL: Low (133 mg)
✓ FAT: Low (19 g)   ✓✓ SODIUM: Very Low (237 mg) **
Exchanges: 5 Meat (extra lean), ¼ Bread, ¼ Veg, 3¾ Fat

† Side dish guidelines are 1/3 of entree guidelines

✓ Low   ✓✓ Very Low

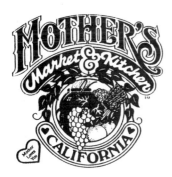

The original Mother's Market & Kitchen was established in 1978, dedicated to the high values of holistic and healthful living. The restaurant offers abundant portions and low prices that complement the beautiful presentation and friendly service. Many loyal fans consider Mother's a second home. They enjoy being able to eat and shop for food at the same place. Now offering "to go" window and outside patio dining. $

Mother's Market & Kitchen
Restaurant, Deli, Fresh Juice & Espresso Bar

Costa Mesa: 225 E. 17th Street (714) 631-4741
Huntington Beach: 19770 Beach Blvd. 963-6667
Irvine: Park Place (Jamboree & Michelson)
Opening summer 1996

BLACKENED TOFU TACOS
with 2 organic corn tortillas, blackened tofu, black beans, and salsa.
✓ CALORIES: Low (464) ✓✓ CHOLESTEROL: None (0 mg)
✓ FAT: Low* (13 g) ✓ SODIUM: Low (535 mg) **
Exchanges: 1¼ Meat (extra lean), 4¾ Bread, 1½ Veg, 3¼ Fat

BOK CHOY BOWL
A bountiful bowlful! Udon noodles, Oriental greens, broccoli, arame seaweed, tofu, onions, sesame oil and spices in a flavorful miso broth.
✓✓ CALORIES: Very Low (305) ✓✓ CHOLESTEROL: None (0 mg)
✓✓ FAT: Very Low* (4 g) SODIUM: High (1110 mg)
Exchanges: ¾ Meat (extra lean), 3¼ Bread, 2½ Veg, 1 Fat

MA'S CHILI
Ma's homemade high protein remedy in an authentic zesty sauce. (14 oz bowl).
✓✓ CALORIES: Very Low (319) ✓✓ CHOLESTEROL: None (0 mg)
✓✓ FAT: Very Low* (2 g) SODIUM: High (1810 mg)
Exchanges: ¾ Meat, ¼ Bread, 7½ Veg

TOFU MUSHROOM MELT - SPECIAL REQUEST
A mouthful! Sauteed tofu, mushroom slices, tomato, lettuce, red onion & sprouts with melted cheese on toasted bread and served with brown rice. Request less oil (1 tsp) & low-fat cheese.
✓ CALORIES: Low (553) ✓✓ CHOLESTEROL: Very Low (6 mg)
✓ FAT: Low (19 g) SODIUM: High (1120 mg)
Exchanges: 3½ Meat, 3¼ Bread, ¾ Veg, 2 Fat

ENERGY SALAD - SPECIAL REQUEST
An energizing combination of sprouts (alfalfa, sunflower & mung bean), atop mixed greenery with avocado slices & raw sunflower seeds. Request reduced portion of avocado (¼ whole). Fat-free and low-fat dressings available (not included in analysis).
✓✓ CALORIES: Very Low (283) ✓✓ CHOLESTEROL: None (0 mg)
✓ FAT: Low* (19 g) ✓✓ SODIUM: Very Low (209 mg) **
Exchanges: 2¼ Veg, 3½ Fat

ORIENTAL STIR-FRY - SPECIAL REQUEST
A medley of fresh Oriental vegetables lightly stir-fried with sesame oil, tamari, fresh ginger and garlic, served with brown rice and almonds.
Request less oil (½ oz) and almonds on the side (almonds not included in analysis).
✓ CALORIES: Low (562) ✓✓ CHOLESTEROL: None (0 mg)
✓ FAT: Low* (17 g) SODIUM: High (1398 mg)
Exchanges: 4½ Bread, 2½ Veg, 2¾ Fat

---

* Primarily unsaturated fat
** If you request no added salt

Mulberry Street

Restaurant & Bar

"A locals' favorite" for the past decade, this cosmopolitan-style restaurant and bar located in the heart of downtown Fullerton has been serving up beautifully prepared home made Italian cuisine and fresh seafood to order. Staffed by a congenial group that will serenade you with one of their original songs on your birthday or special occasion, Mulberry Street is a treat any time of the week. $$

Mulberry Street Restaurant & Bar

114 West Wilshire Ave., Fullerton, CA 92632   (714) 525-1056

BROILED FRESH FISH
with fresh steamed vegetables and pasta marinara. Analysis for halibut; other fish similar.
- ✓ CALORIES: Low (576)
- CHOLESTEROL: Moderate (168 mg)
- ✓✓ FAT: Very Low* (9 g)
- SODIUM: Moderate (676 mg) **

Exchanges: 4½ Meat (extra lean), 3¼ Bread, 2¾ Veg, ¾ Fat

ANGEL HAIR WITH MARINARA SAUCE
- ✓ CALORIES: Low (356)
- ✓✓ CHOLESTEROL: None (0 mg)
- ✓✓ FAT: Very Low* (2 g)
- ✓ SODIUM: Low (493 mg) **

Exchanges: 4½ Bread, 1 Veg

BROILED CHICKEN
with fresh steamed vegetables and pasta marinara.
- ✓ CALORIES: Low (581)
- CHOLESTEROL: Moderate (226 mg)
- ✓✓ FAT: Very Low (9 g)
- SODIUM: Moderate (665 mg) **

Exchanges: 6¾ Meat (extra lean), 3¼ Bread, 2¾ Veg, ¾ Fat

LINGUINI AND FRESH CLAMS IN WHITE SAUCE (2/3 SERVING)
Fresh clams steamed in natural clam broth, white wine, garlic and herbs, over linguini. Analysis is for 2/3 serving.
- ✓ CALORIES: Low (444)
- CHOLESTEROL: Moderate (170 mg)
- ✓✓ FAT: Very Low (7 g)
- ✓ SODIUM: Low (453 mg) **

Exchanges: 2 Meat (extra lean), 4 Bread, ¼ Veg, 1¼ Fat

CHICKEN POMODORO (2/3 SERVING) - SPECIAL REQUEST
Tenderloins of chicken, sauteed in olive oil, garlic, fresh basil, tomatoes and mushrooms and a touch of red wine over fresh linguini. Request less oil (½ oz/full serving). Analysis is for 2/3 serving.
- ✓ CALORIES: Low (544)
- CHOLESTEROL: Moderate (158 mg)
- ✓ FAT: Low (16 g)
- ✓✓ SODIUM: Very Low (86 mg) **

Exchanges: 2¼ Meat (extra lean), 4 Bread, 1 Veg, 2¾ Fat

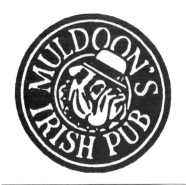

Come experience delicious Irish cooking with a healthy flair. Muldoon's offers fresh fish, specialty salads, award-winning burgers and sandwiches, and homemade Irish delights including chicken, pasta, and Muldoon's famous Irish stew. Muldoon's breakfast menu features a three-to-one omelette with 3 egg whites and 1 egg yolk, filled with garden vegetables and topped with salsa -- low-fat and fantastic! $

Muldoon's Irish Pub & Restaurant
202 Newport Center Dr, Newport Beach, CA 92660
(714) 640-4110

THREE TO ONE OMELETTE - SPECIAL REQUEST
Three egg whites to one yolk omelette filled with fresh garden vegetables & served with salsa. Request less oil (½ oz). Analysis includes fresh fruit and salsa.

✓✓ CALORIES: Very Low (305)   CHOLESTEROL: Moderate (213 mg)
✓ FAT: Low (19 g)   ✓ SODIUM: Low (413 mg) **
Exchanges: 2 Meat, 1 Veg, 1 Fruit, 3½ Fat

GRILLED CHICKEN SALAD - SPECIAL REQUEST
Crisp romaine and red leaf lettuce with slivered China peas, candied pecans, carrots, tomato & a skinless, grilled chicken breast on top. Request dressing on the side (not included in analysis).

✓ CALORIES: Low (523)   CHOLESTEROL: Moderate (152 mg)
✓ FAT: Low (12 g)   ✓✓ SODIUM: Very Low (223 mg) **
Exchanges: 8 Meat (extra lean), 1¾ Bread, 2¼ Veg, 1 Fat

ORIENTAL CHICKEN SALAD - SPECIAL REQUEST
Marinated chicken, Napa curly cabbage, Romaine, Chinese crispy noodles, cucumbers, pecans, sesame seeds & oriental vinaigrette. Request dressing on the side (not included in analysis).

✓ CALORIES: Low (397)   ✓ CHOLESTEROL: Low (87 g)
✓ FAT: Low (17 g)   ✓ SODIUM: Low (433 mg) **
Exchanges: 4½ Meat (extra lean), ½ Bread, 1½ Veg, 2½ Fat

GRILLED FRESH FISH
Analysis shown is for halibut; other fish similar. Served with rosemary potatoes and vegetables (not included in analysis). Request vegetables steamed.

✓ CALORIES: Low (366)   ✓✓ CHOLESTEROL: Very Low (73 mg)
✓ FAT: Low* (19 g)   ✓✓ SODIUM: Very Low (123 mg) **
Exchanges: 4½ Meat (extra lean), 2¾ Fat

RED SNAPPER RANCHERO
Red snapper served on corn tortillas and topped with salsa ranchero.

✓ CALORIES: Low (470)   ✓ CHOLESTEROL: Low (83 mg)
✓ FAT: Low* (18 g)   ✓ SODIUM: Low (397 mg) **
Exchanges: 4¼ Meat (extra lean), 1½ Bread, ½ Veg, 3 Fat

TONY O'CONNOR'S PASTA MARINARA
Fresh tomatoes, basil, garlic & virgin olive oil simmered into a light sauce, tossed with pasta and topped with parmesan.

✓ CALORIES: Low (510)   ✓✓ CHOLESTEROL: Very Low (22 mg)
✓ FAT: Low (14 g)   SODIUM: High (1015 mg) **
Exchanges: 1¾ Meat, 4¼ Bread, ¼ Veg, 1½ Fat

---

* Primarily unsaturated fat
** If you request no added salt

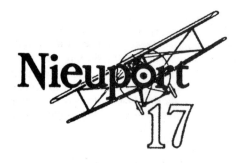

Located on the corner of Irvine Boulevard and Newport Avenue in the city of Tustin, the Nieuport 17 Restaurant is the creation of former Naval Aviator, Bill Bettis. Bill, his Chef James Lane, and General Manager Leslie Stuber have been serving Orange County for twenty-five years. Great continental food in a warm German hunting lodge atmosphere, surrounded by authentic aviation artifacts, photos and paintings, are what make this an outstanding restaurant. $$

Nieuport 17   13051 Newport Ave., Tustin, CA 92680   (714) 731-5130

FRESH CHARBROILED SWORDFISH - SPECIAL REQUEST
with saffron rice and steamed broccoli.
<u>*Request Hollandaise sauce on the side*</u> *(not included in analysis).*
✓ CALORIES: Low (485)   ✓ CHOLESTEROL: Low (78 mg)
✓ FAT: Low* (19 g)   ✓✓ SODIUM: Very Low (261 mg) **
   Exchanges: 4½ Meat (extra lean), 2 Bread, ½ Veg, 2 Fat

FRESH POACHED SALMON - SPECIAL REQUEST
with saffron rice and steamed broccoli.
<u>*Request Hollandaise sauce on the side*</u> *(not included in analysis).*
✓ CALORIES: Low (476)   ✓ CHOLESTEROL: Low (99 mg)
✓ FAT: Low* (18 g)   ✓✓ SODIUM: Very Low (162 mg) **
   Exchanges: 4½ Meat, 2 Bread, ½ Veg, ¼ Fruit, 1¼ Fat

FRESH CHARBROILED HALIBUT - SPECIAL REQUEST
with saffron rice and steamed broccoli.
<u>*Request Hollandaise sauce on the side*</u> *(not included in analysis).*
✓ CALORIES: Low (446)   ✓✓ CHOLESTEROL: Very Low (59 mg)
✓ FAT: Low* (15 g)   ✓✓ SODIUM: Very Low (183 mg) **
   Exchanges: 3½ Meat (extra lean), 2 Bread, ½ Veg, 2 Fat

FRESH VEGETABLE PLATE - SPECIAL REQUEST
Includes fresh vegetables, baked potato (plain), saffron rice, broccoli and zucchini.
<u>*Request sauces and toppings on the side*</u> *(eggplant, sauces & toppings not included in analysis).*
✓ CALORIES: Low (494)   ✓✓ CHOLESTEROL: None (0 mg)
✓✓ FAT: Very Low* (4 g)   ✓✓ SODIUM: Very Low (109 mg) **
      Exchanges: 4¾ Bread, 3 Veg, ½ Fat

SPAGHETTI WITH FRESH TOMATO COULIS
Served with garlic bread (not included in analysis).
✓ CALORIES: Low (418)   ✓✓ CHOLESTEROL: None (0 mg)
✓✓ FAT: Very Low* (9 g)   ✓✓ SODIUM: Very Low (33 mg)
         Exchanges: 3¾ Bread, 2¼ Veg, 1¼ Fat

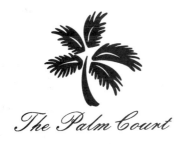

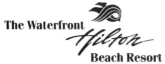

The Palm Court

The Waterfront *Hilton* **Beach Resort**

Whether your travels require a mid-day seaside lunch or an evening meal garnished with golden sunsets, azure seas, and cooling breezes, the Palm Court at the Waterfront Hilton will meet your expectations. This airy room features lilting piano music in the evening and melds the best of Pacific Rim cuisine to more traditional European and Eastern presentations. $$

The Palm Court
at the Waterfront Hilton Beach Resort
21100 Pacific Coast Hwy
Huntington Beach, CA 92648   (714) 960-7873

HERB SEARED TUNA TRIANGLES
Served chilled around rice noodles with a Thai curry sauce.
✓✓ CALORIES: Very Low (282)   ✓ CHOLESTEROL: Low (97 mg)
✓✓ FAT: Very Low (8 g)   ✓✓ SODIUM: Very Low (274 mg) **
Exchanges: 3 Meat (extra lean), 1¼ Bread, ¼ Veg, 1 Fat

FETTUCINE JASMINE
Ginger fettucine with lobster, sea scallops, shiitake mushrooms, snow peas, baby corn, scallions and sesame seeds served in a jasmine tea glaze.
✓ CALORIES: Low (519)   ✓ CHOLESTEROL: Low (92 mg)
✓ FAT: Low (12 g)   SODIUM: Moderate (929 mg) **
Exchanges: 3¼ Meat (extra lean), 3¾ Bread, ¾ Veg, 1¾ Fat

TAHITIAN MAHI MAHI - SPECIAL REQUEST
Teriyaki marinated mahi-mahi broiled and served with volcano shrimp and surrounded with a pineapple orange glaze. Request shrimp grilled. Side dishes vary daily (not included in analysis).
✓ CALORIES: Low (437)   CHOLESTEROL: Moderate (253 mg)
✓ FAT: Low* (16 g)   SODIUM: Moderate (843 mg) **
Exchanges: 4¼ Meat, ¼ Bread, ½ Fruit, 2½ Fat

GRILLED BREAST OF CHICKEN
with mango salsa and garden steamed vegetables. Rice pilaf not included in analysis.
✓ CALORIES: Low (431)   CHOLESTEROL: Moderate (173 mg)
✓✓ FAT: Very Low (8 g)   ✓✓ SODIUM: Very Low (208 mg) **
Exchanges: 9 Meat (extra lean), 1¼ Veg, ¾ Fruit

ANGELO DI CIELO - SPECIAL REQUEST
Angel hair pasta, shrimp, crab claws, peas, fresh herbs, tomato, olive oil and parmesan. Request less oil (½ oz).
✓ CALORIES: Low (594)   ✓ CHOLESTEROL: Low (141 mg)
✓ FAT: Low* (17 g)   ✓✓ SODIUM: Very Low (297 mg) **
Exchanges: 2½ Meat, 4½ Bread, 1 Veg, 2¾ Fat

* Primarily unsaturated fat
** If you request no added salt

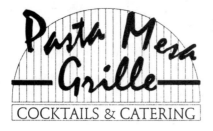

Pasta Mesa Grille is committed to providing our guests with quality food, excellent service and reasonable prices. We are health conscious in the preparation of our foods. Our pastas are made fresh daily and are cholesterol-free. We use low fat milk, low fat cheese, no artificial preservatives or MSG. $$

Pasta Mesa Grille

428 E. 17th Street, Costa Mesa, CA 92627   (714) 642-7488

CAPELLINI BLACK BEAN PASTA
Angel hair pasta, julienne vegetables in a southwest black bean sauce, topped with sour cream and garnished with pine nuts.

✓ CALORIES: Low (406)   ✓✓ CHOLESTEROL: Very Low (6 mg)
✓✓ FAT: Very Low (6 g)   SODIUM: High (2800 mg)
Exchanges: 4 Bread, ¼ Veg, 1 Fat

LINGUINE A LE VONGOLE
Linguine with baby clams, garlic and herbs in olive oil.

✓ CALORIES: Low (571)   ✓ CHOLESTEROL: Low (105 mg)
✓✓ FAT: Very Low* (10 g)   ✓ SODIUM: Low (498 mg) **
Exchanges: 5½ Meat (extra lean), 3¾ Bread, ¼ Veg, 1 Fat

SPAGHETTI A LA MARINARA
✓✓ CALORIES: Very Low (353)   ✓✓ CHOLESTEROL: Very Low (1 mg)
✓✓ FAT: Very Low* (4 g)   ✓✓ SODIUM: Very Low (292 mg) **
Exchanges: 3¾ Bread, 1 Veg, ½ Fat

CAPELLINI AL POMODORO - SPECIAL REQUEST
Angel hair pasta, fresh tomatoes, sun dried tomatoes, black olives, fresh basil and garlic in olive oil. <u>*Request less oil*</u> *(½ oz).*

✓ CALORIES: Low (459)   ✓✓ CHOLESTEROL: None (0 mg)
✓ FAT: Low* (17 g)   ✓ SODIUM: Low (434 mg) **
Exchanges: 3¾ Bread, 1½ Veg, 2¾ Fat

POLLO CACCIATORE - SPECIAL REQUEST
Chicken breast baked with vegetables and tomato sauce, and served with linguine and marinara sauce. <u>*Request less oil*</u> *(½ oz).*

✓ CALORIES: Low (505)   ✓ CHOLESTEROL: Low (121 mg)
✓ FAT: Low (20 g)   ✓✓ SODIUM: Very Low (227 mg) **
Exchanges: 6¼ Meat (extra lean), 1¼ Bread, 1¼ Veg, 3 Fat

† Side dish guidelines are 1/3 of entree guidelines

✓ Low   ✓✓ Very Low

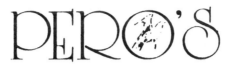

PERO'S

Located in Sea Cliff Village, our charming restaurant will remind you of a coastal bistro you might find in Italy. As you stroll past the herb garden in the unique glass entrance, you are greeted with a friendly welcome. Pero's has been in this location for 16 years, and its history of fabulous food is noted by the many awards and faithful customers. Enjoy the best of Italy for breakfast, lunch or dinner. $$

Pero's
Sea Cliff Village, 2221 North Main, Huntington Beach, CA 92648   (714) 960-7764

FRESH FISH - SPECIAL REQUEST
Analysis is for halibut (other fish similar) and carrots. Request sauce on the side (not included in analysis) and side dish of Spaghetti with Tomato Sauce (analysis below).
- ✓ CALORIES: Low (389)
- ✓ FAT: Low (16 g)
- ✓ CHOLESTEROL: Low (83 mg)
- ✓✓ SODIUM: Very Low (201 mg) **

Exchanges: 4½ Meat (extra lean), 2¼ Veg, 2 Fat

SPAGHETTI AND TOMATO SAUCE
- ✓ CALORIES: Low (427)
- ✓✓ FAT: Very Low* (7 g)
- ✓✓ CHOLESTEROL: None (0 mg)
- SODIUM: Moderate (769 mg) **

Exchanges: 4¼ Bread, 2 Veg, ¼ Fruit, 1¼ Fat

FETTUCCINE WITH RED SHRIMP SAUCE (2/3 SERVING)
- ✓ CALORIES: Low (445)
- ✓ FAT: Low (12 g)
- CHOLESTEROL: Moderate (193 mg)
- SODIUM: Moderate (592 mg) **

Exchanges: 1½ Meat (extra lean), 2¾ Bread, ¾ Veg, 2 Fat

FETTUCCINE PRIMAVERA (2/3 SERVING) - SPECIAL REQUEST
Fettuccine tossed in a marinara sauce with broccoli, cauliflower, mushrooms, carrots and yams. Request no Alfredo in the marinara sauce.
- ✓ CALORIES: Low (479)
- ✓ FAT: Low* (20 g)
- ✓✓ CHOLESTEROL: None (0 mg)
- SODIUM: Moderate (678 mg) **

Exchanges: 2¾ Bread, 4 Veg, 3½ Fat

SEAFOOD LINGUINE (2/3 SERVING) - SPECIAL REQUEST
Scallops, shrimp and clams tossed in a marinara sauce. Request less butter (½ oz) and no Alfredo in the marinara sauce.
- ✓ CALORIES: Low (499)
- ✓ FAT: Low (16 g)
- ✓ CHOLESTEROL: Low (150 mg)
- ✓ SODIUM: Low (583 mg) **

Exchanges: 2¾ Meat (extra lean), 2¾ Bread, 1¾ Veg, 2½ Fat

SIDE DISH: SPAGHETTI WITH TOMATO SAUCE[†]
- CALORIES: Moderate (220)
- ✓✓ FAT: Very Low* (3 g)
- ✓✓ CHOLESTEROL: None (0 mg)
- SODIUM: Moderate (289 mg) **

Exchanges: 2 Bread, ¾ Veg, ½ Fat

---

* Primarily unsaturated fat
** If you request no added salt

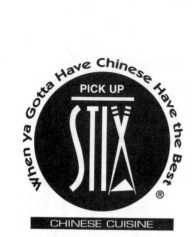

Pick Up Stix

Anaheim Hills: 5576 E. Santa Ana Cyn Rd (714) 974-9777
Irvine: 5365 Alton Parkway (714) 786-7849
Laguna Niguel: 27000 Alicia Pkwy (714) 643-0779
Laguna Niguel: 30012 Crown Valley Pkwy (714) 495-5730
Newport Beach: 1112 Irvine Avenue (714) 650-7849
Newport Beach: 1614 San Miguel Drive (714) 759-8200
Placentia: 187 E. Yorba Linda Blvd (714) 524-8000
San Clemente: 415 Avenida Pico (714) 492-1226
Tustin: 13289 Jamboree Road (714) 573-0992
Rancho Santa Margarita: (714) 589-0522
    31441 Santa Margarita Pkwy

Welcome to Pick Up Stix Chinese Cuisine -- a unique dining experience. Along with many of the traditional Asian recipes, you will find numerous culinary creations and combinations of the best quality foods and specialty spices and herbs. All of our food is prepared without the usual heavy and/or salty sauces and without the use of MSG. $

CHINESE CHICKEN SALAD
Fresh greens with oven-roasted breast of chicken, served with our special dressing and topped with sunflower seeds and Chinese croutons. Analysis is for a full serving.
- ✓ CALORIES: Low (359)
- ✓ FAT: Low (15 g)
- ✓ CHOLESTEROL: Low (94 mg)
- ✓ SODIUM: Low (331 mg) **

Exchanges: 4½ Meat (extra lean), ½ Bread, 1 Veg, 2 Fat

GARLIC CHICKEN (½ SERVING)
Chicken wok'd with broccoli, onions, mushrooms and water chestnuts in our special garlic sauce. Analysis is for ½ serving and ½ cup steamed rice.
- ✓ CALORIES: Low (413)
- ✓✓ FAT: Very Low (10 g)
- ✓ CHOLESTEROL: Low (109 mg)
- SODIUM: High (1232 mg)

Exchanges: 4¼ Meat, 2 Bread, 1¾ Veg

SEASONAL VEGETABLES (½ SERVING)
A colorful array of fresh vegetables skillfully stir-sauteed in a light sauce to bring out their natural flavors. Analysis is for ½ serving of vegetables and ½ cup steamed rice.
- ✓✓ CALORIES: Very Low (226)
- ✓✓ FAT: Very Low* (4 g)
- ✓✓ CHOLESTEROL: None (0 mg)
- ✓ SODIUM: Low (367 mg) **

Exchanges: 1¾ Bread, 2¾ Veg, ¾ Fat

MONGOLIAN BEEF (½ SERVING)
Tender beef, wok'd with green and white onions and served on a bed of rice noodles (noodles not included in analysis). Analysis is for ½ serving and ½ cup steamed rice.
- ✓ CALORIES: Low (374)
- ✓ FAT: Low (11 g)
- ✓✓ CHOLESTEROL: Very Low (48 mg)
- SODIUM: High (1069 mg)

Exchanges: 3¾ Meat, 2 Bread, ¾ Veg, ½ Fat

HOUSE SPECIAL CHICKEN (½ SERVING)
Our most popular dish. Tender diced chicken served in a dark sauce of white wine, ginger, soy and green onions with a dash of white pepper. Analysis is for ½ serving and ½ cup steamed rice.
- ✓ CALORIES: Low (575)
- ✓ FAT: Low (20 g)
- CHOLESTEROL: Moderate (191 mg)
- SODIUM: High (1217 mg)

Exchanges: 7½ Meat, 2¼ Bread, ½ Fat

✓ Low   ✓✓ Very Low

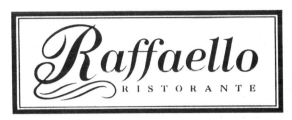

Winner of the prestigious Restaurant Writers Award, Raffaello Ristorante remains ever so popular in the city of Orange. Unique hot & cold appetizers, fresh salads, custom pastas, chicken, veal, seafood and meats are among the dining pleasures awaiting those who step into the beautiful modern Mediterranean dining room. Located right off the Costa Mesa (55) Freeway at Tustin. $$

Raffaello Ristorante 1998 N. Tustin Ave, Orange, CA 92665 (714) 283-8230

PIZZA RAFFAELLO (½ PIZZA)

with fresh tomatoes, olive oil, dash of garlic, fresh basil and no cheese. Analysis is for ½ pizza.

✓ CALORIES: Low (547) ✓✓ CHOLESTEROL: None (0 mg)
✓ FAT: Low* (18 g) SODIUM: High (1057 mg)
Exchanges: 4¾ Bread, 1¼ Veg, 3¼ Fat

SALMONE ALLA CALABRESE - SPECIAL REQUEST

Salmon steaks perfectly grilled and topped with fresh tomatoes, fresh herbs, lemon & extra virgin olive oil. Request less oil (½ Tbs). Analysis is for lunch portion; dinner portion slightly higher.

✓ CALORIES: Low (371) ✓ CHOLESTEROL: Low (91 mg)
✓ FAT: Low* (19 g) SODIUM: Moderate (948 mg) **
Exchanges: 4¼ Meat, 1¼ Veg, 1½ Fat

LINGUINE ALLE VONGOLE WITH WHITE SAUCE (2/3 SERVING) -

SPECIAL REQUEST *sauteed with fresh clams, white wine, garlic & fresh herbs. Request less oil (1 Tbs/full serving). Analysis is for 2/3 of a large serving.*

✓ CALORIES: Low (518) ✓✓ CHOLESTEROL: Very Low (64 mg)
✓ FAT: Low* (12 g) SODIUM: Moderate (673 mg) **
Exchanges: 3¼ Meat (extra lean), 3½ Bread, 1 Veg, 1¾ Fat

LINGUINE MARI E MONTI (2/3 SERVING) - SPECIAL REQUEST

with fresh shrimp, calamari and porcini mushrooms sauteed with garlic in a fresh tomato sauce. Request less oil (1 Tbs/full serving). Analysis is for 2/3 of a large serving.

✓ CALORIES: Low (582) CHOLESTEROL: Moderate (290 mg)
✓ FAT: Low* (15 g) SODIUM: Moderate (764 mg) **
Exchanges: 2½ Meat (extra lean), 3½ Bread, 1¼ Veg, 2¼ Fat

POLLO CALABRESE - SPECIAL REQUEST

Grilled boneless breast of chicken topped with fresh tomatoes, fresh herbs, lemon and extra virgin olive oil. Request less oil (½ Tbs).

✓ CALORIES: Low (599) CHOLESTEROL: Moderate (238 mg)
✓ FAT: Low (18 g) SODIUM: High (1080 mg)
Exchanges: 12½ Meat (extra lean), 1¼ Veg, 1½ Fat

---

* Primarily unsaturated fat
** If you request no added salt

Healthy Dining in Orange County **97**

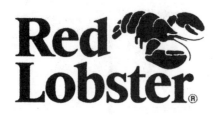

At Red Lobster, we strive everyday to offer gracious, personalized service. Our approach is simple...treat customers in our restaurant as we would guests in our home. Our seafood is the finest, especially our sensible "Lighthouse Selections," where 30% or less of the calories are from fat. We look forward to your visit, where a myriad of succulent choices awaits you. $$

Red Lobster locations:

Anaheim: 1199 N. Euclid Ave. (Just south of 91 Freeway on Euclid Ave.)	(714) 778-5000
Brea: 250 Brea Mall Way (One mile north of Imperial Hwy)	(714) 529-0632
El Toro: 23694 El Toro Rd. (Two blocks east of I-5 in Saddleback Valley Plaza)	(714) 586-3474
Garden Grove: 12892 Harbor Blvd. (One block north of Garden Grove Blvd)	(714) 638-9500
La Palma: 50 Center Pointe (Four miles east of I-5)	(714) 562-9086
Seal Beach: 620 Pacific Coast Hwy. (Just south of Long Beach Marina)	(310) 594-9777

LIVE MAINE LOBSTER
A real Northeastern delicacy. Butter not included in analysis.
- ✓✓ CALORIES: Very Low (190)
- ✓ CHOLESTEROL: Low (125 mg)
- ✓✓ FAT: Very Low* (1½ g)
- SODIUM: Moderate (680 mg) **

SNOW CRAB LEGS
Steamed and served with hot melted butter. Butter not included in analysis.
- ✓✓ CALORIES: Very Low (140)
- ✓ CHOLESTEROL: Low (115 mg)
- ✓✓ FAT: Very Low* (2 g)
- ✓ SODIUM: Low (330 mg) **

BROILED ROCK LOBSTER TAIL
Lightly seasoned and broiled. Butter not included in analysis.
- ✓✓ CALORIES: Very Low (200)
- ✓ CHOLESTEROL: Low (100 mg)
- ✓✓ FAT: Very Low* (6 g)
- SODIUM: Moderate (680 mg) **

FRESH KING SALMON
Guaranteed to be the finest fresh fish available. Analysis for 5 oz lunch portion.
- ✓✓ CALORIES: Very Low (250)
- ✓ CHOLESTEROL: Low (95 mg)
- ✓ FAT: Low* (15 g)
- ✓✓ SODIUM: Very Low (70 mg) **

BAKED COD
A delicate fillet lightly seasoned and baked.
- ✓ CALORIES: Low (450)
- ✓ CHOLESTEROL: Low (100 mg)
- ✓✓ FAT: Very Low* (10 g)
- SODIUM: High (1490 mg)

GARLIC HERB-SEARED CHICKEN - SPECIAL REQUEST
Marinated in a garlic marinade and grilled to a golden brown. <u>Request skin removed</u>.
- ✓ CALORIES: Low (500)
- ✓ CHOLESTEROL: Low (130 mg)
- ✓✓ FAT: Very Low (10 g)
- SODIUM: High (1150 mg)

Nutrition Information supplied by Red Lobster®

† Side dish guidelines are 1/3 of entree guidelines

✓ Low ✓✓ Very Low

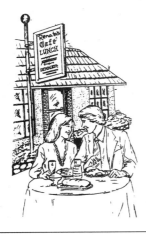

Our goal is to keep tastes, character, and traditions intact -- bringing you the flavors of Italy in all their glory. We try to be as original as possible, keeping recipes authentic, using the best and freshest products in the market, and making our pasta the old-fashioned way. We put all our knowledge and love in every dish we serve you. Buon Appetito! $$

Renata's Caffé Italiano

227 East Chapman Avenue
Orange, CA 92666   (714) 771-4740

VERDURA ALLA GRIGLIA
A mix of grilled vegetables marinated in balsamic vinegar.
Served with Pasta Marinara (analysis below).
✓✓ CALORIES: Very Low (249)   ✓✓ CHOLESTEROL: None (0 mg)
✓ FAT: Low* (15 g)   SODIUM: High (1198 mg)
Exchanges: ½ Bread, 2 Veg, 2¾ Fat

PESCE DEL GIORNO FLORENTINE
Grilled fish with fresh steamed spinach. Analysis is for sea bass, other fish similar. Served with Pasta Marinara (analysis below).
✓✓ CALORIES: Very Low (350)   ✓ CHOLESTEROL: Low (108 mg)
✓ FAT: Low* (12 g)   SODIUM: High (1008 mg)
Exchanges: 7 Meat (extra lean), 1¼ Veg, 1¼ Fat

PENNE ALL'ARRABBIATA
Penne with spicy marinara sauce.
✓ CALORIES: Low (583)   ✓✓ CHOLESTEROL: None (0 mg)
✓ FAT: Low* (16 g)   ✓ SODIUM: Low (375 mg) **
Exchanges: 5¼ Bread, 2¾ Veg, 2¾ Fat

CAPELLINI PRIMAVERA
Angel hair pasta with fresh steamed vegetables, fresh tomatoes, garlic and onions.
✓ CALORIES: Low (535)   ✓✓ CHOLESTEROL: None (0 mg)
✓ FAT: Low* (15 g)   ✓✓ SODIUM: Very Low (51 mg) **
Exchanges: 4¼ Bread, 2¾ Veg, 2¾ Fat

SIDE DISH: PASTA MARINARA†
CALORIES: Moderate (291)   ✓✓ CHOLESTEROL: None (0 mg)
FAT: Moderate* (8 g)   ✓ SODIUM: Low (187 mg) **
Exchanges: 2½ Bread, 1¼ Veg, 1¼ Fat

---

* Primarily unsaturated fat
** If you request no added salt

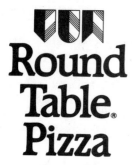

Round Table Pizza not only makes the freshest, best-tasting, real pizza in town, it's also good for you. Our line of healthier Saluté Pizzas are great tasting, with less fat and more fresh toppings. It's the perfect food for today's busy lifestyles. We make our pizzas with a variety of sauces, a blend of three real cheeses, superior meats, the freshest vegetables, and dough made fresh in our restaurants. Round Table Pizza offers 25 locations in Orange County for your convenience. $

Round Table Pizza

Locations in Anaheim, Brea, Costa Mesa, Cypress, Diamond Bar, Fullerton, Fountain Valley, Garden Grove, Huntington Beach, Irvine, La Mirada, Laguna Hills, Laguna Niguel, Mission Viejo, San Clemente, Santa Ana, Tustin, Westminster & Yorba Linda.

Analyses below are for thin crust pizza; pan crust adds approx. ½ g fat & 50 calories per slice.

GUINEVERE'S GARDEN DELIGHT PIZZA (2 SLICES)
Cheese, mushrooms, olives, fresh tomatoes, onions & green peppers. Analysis for 2 slices large pizza.
- ✓✓ CALORIES: Very Low (300)
- ✓ FAT: Low (11.2 g)
- ✓✓ CHOLESTEROL: Very Low (30 mg)
- ✓ SODIUM: Low (500 mg)

GOURMET VEGGIE PIZZA (2 SLICES)
Creamy garlic sauce, three cheeses, artichoke hearts, zucchini, spinach, mushrooms, tomatoes, red & green onions, Italian herb seasoning, and lots of chopped garlic. Analysis for 2 slices large pizza.
- ✓✓ CALORIES: Very Low (320)
- ✓ FAT: Low (13 g)
- ✓✓ CHOLESTEROL: Very Low (30 mg)
- ✓ SODIUM: Low (400 mg)

CHICKEN & GARLIC GOURMET PIZZA (2 SLICES)
Creamy garlic sauce, three cheeses, chunks of chicken, mushrooms, tomatoes, red & green onions, Italian herb seasoning & lots of chopped garlic. Analysis for 2 slices large pizza.
- ✓✓ CALORIES: Very Low (340)
- ✓ FAT: Low (14.4 g)
- ✓✓ CHOLESTEROL: Very Low (50 mg)
- ✓ SODIUM: Low (560 mg)

SALUTÉ CASHEW CHICKEN PIZZA (2 SLICES)
Sweet & spicy Oriental chili sauce, 3 cheeses, roasted chicken, roasted cashews, pineapple, zucchini, green peppers, carrots, yellow onions, garlic, Roma tomatoes & green onions. Analysis for 2 slices large pizza.
- ✓✓ CALORIES: Very Low (300)
- ✓✓ FAT: Very Low (8.2 g)
- ✓✓ CHOLESTEROL: Very Low (30 mg)
- ✓ SODIUM: Low (480 mg)

SALUTÉ VEGGIE PIZZA (2 SLICES)
Creamy garlic sauce, three cheeses, artichoke hearts, zucchini, roasted red & green peppers, mushrooms, red onions, spinach, green onions, Roma tomatoes, roasted garlic, Italian herb seasoning & shredded Parmesan cheese. Analysis for 2 slices large pizza.
- ✓✓ CALORIES: Very Low (280)
- ✓✓ FAT: Very Low (9.4 g)
- ✓✓ CHOLESTEROL: Very Low (20 mg)
- ✓ SODIUM: Low (340 mg)

Nutrition information supplied by Round Table Pizza.

✓ Low   ✓✓ Very Low

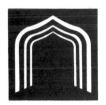

ROYAL KHYBER
Cuisine of India

*Royal Khyber features the finest in Indian cuisine.
An intimate atmosphere and spectacularly presented
dishes create an ultimate dining experience.* $$

Royal Khyber Cuisine of India
1000 Bristol Street North, Newport Beach, CA 92660 (714) 752-5200

DAL MAKHANI
Lentils and beans in a special blend of spices.
✓✓ CALORIES: Very Low (198)   ✓✓ CHOLESTEROL: None (0 mg)
✓✓ FAT: Very Low* (7 g)   ✓✓ SODIUM: Very Low (58 mg) **
Exchanges: ¾ Meat (extra lean), 1¼ Bread, ¾ Veg, 1¼ Fat

TANDOORI SWORDFISH TIKKA
*Cubed fish, marinated in yogurt and mild spices
and baked in a hot Tandoor clay oven.*
✓✓ CALORIES: Very Low (298)   ✓ CHOLESTEROL: Low (98 mg)
✓ FAT: Low* (11 g)   ✓✓ SODIUM: Very Low (295 mg) **
Exchanges: 5¼ Meat, ¼ Fat

KARAHI CHICKEN
Chicken prepared with curry of tomatoes, olive oil and herbs. Choose mild, medium or hot.
✓ CALORIES: Low (408)   CHOLESTEROL: Moderate (152 mg)
✓ FAT: Low (14 g)   ✓✓ SODIUM: Very Low (150 mg) **
Exchanges: 8 Meat (extra lean), 1½ Veg, 1¼ Fat

KARAHI SHRIMP
Shrimp prepared with curry of tomatoes, olive oil and herbs. Choose mild, medium or hot.
✓✓ CALORIES: Very Low (261)   CHOLESTEROL: Moderate (290 mg)
✓✓ FAT: Very Low* (9 g)   ✓ SODIUM: Low (347 mg) **
Exchanges: 2¾ Meat (extra lean), 1½ Veg, 1¼ Fat

TANDOORI CHICKEN TIKKA
*A succulent boneless breast of chicken, marinated in yogurt
and mild spices and baked in a hot Tandoor clay oven.*
✓ CALORIES: Low (339)   CHOLESTEROL: Moderate (173 mg)
✓✓ FAT: Very Low (7 g)   ✓✓ SODIUM: Very Low (160 mg) **
Exchanges: 9 Meat (extra lean)

ALOO GOBI - SPECIAL REQUEST
Cauliflower and potatoes in mild herbs and spices. <u>Request less oil (½ oz)</u>.
✓✓ CALORIES: Very Low (292)   ✓✓ CHOLESTEROL: None (0 mg)
✓ FAT: Low* (15 g)   ✓✓ SODIUM: Very Low (35 mg) **
Exchanges: 1½ Bread, 2¼ Veg, 2¾ Fat

---

* Primarily unsaturated fat
** If you request no added salt

Royal Thai

Cuisine

*Royal Thai -- award-winning exotic cuisine
and beautiful ambience. Extensive menu features
authentic Thai dishes from recipes handed down
through the Tila family for generations. You'll
enjoy a wide selection of delights to please your
taste, either hot or mild. Let Royal Thai cater
to you -- there's something to please everyone. $*

Royal Thai Cuisine

4001 W. Pacific Coast Hwy, Newport Beach, CA 92663   (714) 645-THAI
1750 S. Coast Highway, Laguna Beach, CA 92651   (714) 494-THAI

NAKED SHRIMP (½ SERVING)
*Grilled, medium rare shrimp seasoned with lime, nampla and chili mingled
with lemon grass (hot and spicy). Analysis is for ½ serving.*
✓✓ CALORIES: Very Low (347)   CHOLESTEROL: Moderate (368 mg)
✓✓ FAT: Very Low* (4 g)   SODIUM: High (2368 mg)
　　　　Exchanges: 3½ Meat (extra lean), 1½ Bread, 1¼ Veg, ¼ Fruit

HOT BASIL WITH OYSTER MUSHROOMS (½ SERVING) - SPECIAL REQUEST
*with bell peppers, onions, mushrooms, chili and garlic sauce (hot and spicy).
<u>Request less oil</u> (2 Tbs/full serving). Analysis is for ½ serving.*
✓✓ CALORIES: Very Low (250)   ✓✓ CHOLESTEROL: Very Low (2 mg)
✓ FAT: Low* (15 g)   SODIUM: Moderate (749 mg)**
　　　　Exchanges: ¼ Bread, 4¼ Veg, 2¾ Fat

ROYAL YACHT (½ SERVING)
*A combination of seafood carefully prepared with cabbage, celery and silver noodles,
blended with spices, and served in a royal yacht. Analysis is for ½ serving.*
✓ CALORIES: Low (497)   ✓ CHOLESTEROL: Low (141 mg)
✓ FAT: Low* (15 g)   SODIUM: High (1421 mg)
　　　　Exchanges: 1½ Meat, 3¾ Bread, 2 Veg, 2¾ Fat

CHICKEN WITH EGGPLANT & BAMBOO SHOOTS (½ SERVING) - SPECIAL REQUEST
*Asian eggplant, chicken and bamboo shoots in sweet basil and chili sauce.
<u>Request less oil</u> (2 Tbs/full serving). Analysis is for ½ serving.*
✓ CALORIES: Low (391)   ✓ CHOLESTEROL: Low (109 mg)
✓ FAT: Low (20 g)   ✓ SODIUM: Low (549 mg)**
　　　　Exchanges: 5½ Meat (extra lean), ¼ Bread, 1 Veg, 2¾ Fat

STEAMED FRESH CATCH OF THE DAY WITH SPICY THAI SAUCE
<u>Request steamed</u> for no added oil. Analysis is for sea bass; other fish similar.
✓ CALORIES: Low (506)   ✓ CHOLESTEROL: Low (118 mg)
✓✓ FAT: Very Low* (7 g)   SODIUM: High (3921 mg)
　　　　Exchanges: 5 Meat (extra lean), 1¾ Bread, 4¼ Veg

Ruby's Diner with 14 Orange County locations to serve you!

The Original, Balboa Pier	(714) 675-7829
2305 E. Coast Hwy, Corona del Mar	(714) 673-7829
3333 Bear Street, Costa Mesa	(714) 662-7829
1301 S. Harbor Blvd., Fullerton	(714) 871-7829
4602 Barranca Pkwy, Irvine	(714) 552-7829
30622 S. Coast Hwy, Laguna Beach	(714) 497-7829
24155 Laguna Hills Mall, Laguna Hills	(714) 588-7829
27762 Vista Del Lago, Mission Viejo	(714) 770-7829
3000 W. Coast Hwy., Newport Beach	(714) 631-7829
2800 N. Main St., Main Place Mall, Santa Ana	(714) 836-7829
Seal Beach Pier, Seal Beach	(310) 431-7829
13102 Newport Ave., Tustin	(714) 838-7829
21450 Yorba Linda Blvd., Yorba Linda	(714) 779-7829
31781 Camino Capistrano, San Juan Capistrano	(714) 496-7829

Additional locations in LA & San Diego Counties. More coming soon!

Ruby's Diner is the authentic 40's diner in Southern California! Step back in time to 40's memorabilia, gleaming red and white interiors and friendly, courteous service. We offer items to please every palate, including a variety of salads, sandwiches, and home style breakfasts. Swing by Ruby's today and experience great food & great service with a 40's flair. $

VEGGIE RUBYBURGER - SPECIAL REQUEST
with a tasty vegetable, rice, oats and wheat patty. Request no margarine and Ruby sauce on the side (not included in analysis).
- ✓ CALORIES: Low (384)
- ✓✓ CHOLESTEROL: Very Low (8 mg)
- ✓✓ FAT: Very Low* (7 g)
- SODIUM: Moderate (664 mg) **

Exchanges: ½ Meat, 4 Bread, ¼ Veg, 1¼ Fat

CHICKEN RUBYBURGER - SPECIAL REQUEST
with a tender, boneless, skinless chicken breast. Request no margarine or mayonnaise.
- ✓ CALORIES: Low (466)
- ✓ CHOLESTEROL: Low (130 mg)
- ✓✓ FAT: Very Low (9 g)
- ✓ SODIUM: Low (516 mg) **

Exchanges: 6¾ Meat (extra lean), 2¼ Bread, ¼ Veg, ¾ Fat

TURKEY RUBYBURGER - SPECIAL REQUEST
with a full 1/3 lb. of lean ground turkey.
Request no margarine and Ruby sauce on the side (not included in analysis).
- ✓ CALORIES: Low (427)
- ✓✓ CHOLESTEROL: Very Low (64 mg)
- ✓ FAT: Low (17 g)
- ✓ SODIUM: Low (501 mg) **

Exchanges: 3¼ Meat, 2¼ Bread, ¼ Veg, 1¼ Fat

ROAST TURKEY BREAST SANDWICH - SPECIAL REQUEST
served with lettuce & cranberry sauce on a soft RubyRoll. Just like Thanksgiving!
Request no margarine or mayonnaise.
- ✓ CALORIES: Low (475)
- ✓ CHOLESTEROL: Low (118 mg)
- ✓✓ FAT: Very Low (3 g)
- ✓ SODIUM: Low (523 mg) **

Exchanges: 6¼ Meat (extra lean), 2½ Bread, 1½ Fruit, ¼ Fat

CHINESE CHICKEN SALAD - SPECIAL REQUEST
Fresh greens, crisp celery, green onion, red bell pepper, rice noodles & a tender grilled chicken breast. Request sesame dressing on the side (not included in analysis).
- ✓ CALORIES: Low (421)
- ✓ CHOLESTEROL: Low (149 mg)
- ✓ FAT: Low (11 g)
- SODIUM: Moderate (828 mg) **

Exchanges: 7 Meat (extra lean), ½ Bread, 1½ Veg, ¾ Fat

---

* Primarily unsaturated fat
** If you request no added salt

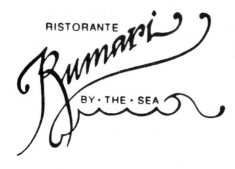

RISTORANTE

Rumari

BY·THE·SEA

Rumari Ristorante emanates a warm and cozy dining atmosphere that features exquisite, award-winning Italian cuisine, prepared by Mamma Bina and her four sons. The quiet elegance of Laguna Beach serves as a beginning to a menu which includes a variety of Northern and Southern dishes and specialties which include black linguini seafood, veal, lobster ravioli, and rolled eggplant stuffed with spaghetti. Rumari also offers an extensive Italian wine list and cocktails. $$

Rumari   1826 South Coast Hwy, Laguna Beach, CA 92651   (714) 494-0400

SPAGHETTI SIRACUSANA
*Thin spaghetti pasta tossed with eggplant, roasted peppers,
onions and romano cheese, in a tomato sauce.*
✓ CALORIES: Low (540)   ✓✓ CHOLESTEROL: Very Low (7 mg)
✓ FAT: Low* (19 g)   ✓✓ SODIUM: Very Low (236 mg) **
        Exchanges: ¼ Meat, 4½ Bread, 1½ Veg, 3¼ Fat

INVOLTINI DI MELANZANE E SPAGHETTI
Grilled eggplant filled with spaghetti and served in a light tomato sauce.
✓ CALORIES: Low (544)   ✓✓ CHOLESTEROL: Very Low (6 mg)
✓ FAT: Low* (19 g)   ✓✓ SODIUM: Very Low (277 mg) **
        Exchanges: ¼ Meat, 4¾ Bread, ¾ Veg, 3¼ Fat

VERMICELLI PICCHIO PACCHIO - SPECIAL REQUEST
*Angel hair pasta with fresh tomatoes, sun-dried tomatoes, basil,
garlic and olive oil. Request less oil (½ oz).*
✓ CALORIES: Low (546)   ✓✓ CHOLESTEROL: None (0 mg)
✓ FAT: Low* (16 g)   ✓✓ SODIUM: Very Low (46 mg) **
        Exchanges: 4¼ Bread, 1 Veg, 2¾ Fat

POLLO ALLA GRIGLIA CON ERBE - SPECIAL REQUEST
*Grilled boneless chicken breast with lemon, oil, garlic and herbs. Request less
oil (½ oz) and vegetables grilled. Potatoes not included in analysis.*
✓ CALORIES: Low (483)   CHOLESTEROL: Moderate (152 mg)
✓ FAT: Low (20 g)   ✓✓ SODIUM: Very Low (165 mg) **
        Exchanges: 8 Meat (extra lean), 1½ Veg, ½ Fruit, 2¾ Fat

SCAMPI ALLA GRIGLIA - SPECIAL REQUEST
Request less oil (½ oz) and vegetables grilled. Potatoes not included in analysis.
✓ CALORIES: Low (370)   CHOLESTEROL: (394 mg)
✓ FAT: Low* (16 g)   ✓ SODIUM: Low (476 mg) **
        Exchanges: 3¾ Meat (extra lean), 1¼ Veg, ¼ Fruit, 2¾ Fat

† Side dish guidelines are 1/3 of entree guidelines
✓ Low   ✓✓ Very Low

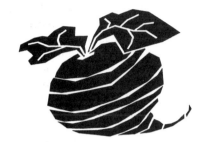

RUTABÉGORZ

At Rutabégorz, one of Orange County's oldest coffee houses, the emphasis has always been on fresh ingredients and simple preparation. It is the perfect place to get a truly phenomenal salad. But if you are not in a salad mood, there are lots of hot entrees, sandwiches, and soups, many of which are vegetarian. Cash, cheques, VISA and MasterCard gladly accepted. $

Rutabégorz

158 West Main Street, Tustin, CA (714) 731-9807
211 North Pomona, Fullerton, CA (714) 738-9339
4610 Barranca Parkway, Irvine, CA (714) 733-1444

VEGETARIAN CHILI (1 CUP)
Beans, soy protein and veggies. Cheese, crackers and garnishes not included in analysis.
✓✓ CALORIES: Very Low (171)   ✓✓ CHOLESTEROL: Very Low (11 mg)
✓✓ FAT: Very Low* (5 g)   SODIUM: High (1004 mg)
Exchanges: ¼ Meat, 1¼ Bread, ½ Veg, ¾ Fat

YOU TURKEY SANDWICH - SPECIAL REQUEST
Turkey breast, lettuce & tomatoes on squaw bread. Request no cheese.
Low-fat mayo, mustard and fruit served on the side (not included in analysis).
✓ CALORIES: Low (547)   ✓ CHOLESTEROL: Low (142 mg)
✓✓ FAT: Very Low (7 g)   SODIUM: Moderate (835 mg) **
Exchanges: 7½ Meat (extra lean), 3 Bread, 1¼ Veg, ¾ Fat

VEGGIE SURPRISE - SPECIAL REQUEST
A combo of fresh veggies and sunflower seeds on top a mound of rice pilaf.
Request no cheese. Squaw bread, salsa and fruit not included in analysis.
✓ CALORIES: Low (588)   ✓✓ CHOLESTEROL: None (0 mg)
✓ FAT: Low* (20 g)   ✓✓ SODIUM: Very Low (111 mg) **
Exchanges: 4¼ Bread, 3½ Veg, 3¼ Fat

CURRY CHICKEN SALAD - SPECIAL REQUEST
Chicken, peanuts, all the veggies and greens served with a whole wheat tortilla.
Request less peanuts (½ oz) and dressing on the side (dressing not included in analysis).
✓ CALORIES: Low (527)   ✓ CHOLESTEROL: Low (108 mg)
✓ FAT: Low (13 g)   ✓ SODIUM: Low (367 mg) **
Exchanges: 6 Meat, 6½ Veg, 1 Bread, 1¼ Fat

RICE A RUTA'S - SPECIAL REQUEST
A mixture of shrimp and chicken and veggies atop a bed of rice. Request no
crunchy noodles. Cheese bread, fruit and salsa not included in analysis.
CALORIES: Moderate (751)   CHOLESTEROL: Moderate (218 mg)
✓ FAT: Low (12 g)   ✓ SODIUM: Low (537 mg) **
Exchanges: 5¾ Meat, 5¾ Bread, 2 Veg

CHICKEN RICE VEGETABLE SOUP†
Chicken, lots o' veggies and rice.
✓✓ CALORIES: Very Low (79)   ✓✓ CHOLESTEROL: Very Low (16 mg)
✓✓ FAT: Very Low (2 g)   SODIUM: High (928 mg)
Exchanges: ¾ Meat, ¼ Bread, ¾ Veg

---

* Primarily unsaturated fat
** If you request no added salt

Sapori

Sapori is truly a taste of Italy...authentic in every detail from its casual, friendly ambiance to its delightful food and service. At Sapori you'll find sensational housemade pastas, uniquely prepared fresh fish, brick oven pizzas, delicate veal specialties, innovative daily specials, award-winning desserts and a fine selection of Italian and California wines. $$

Sapori Ristorante   1080 Bayside Dr, Newport Beach, CA 92660   (714) 644-4220
Sapori Trattoria   2991 El Camino Real, Tustin, CA 92680   (714) 731-7480

PIZZA ARLECCHINO (½ PIZZA)
with sundried tomatoes, artichoke hearts, chicken, fresh basil and fresh mozzarella. Analysis is for ½ pizza.
- ✓ CALORIES: Low (445)   ✓✓ CHOLESTEROL: Very Low (20 mg)
- ✓ FAT: Low (16 g)   SODIUM: Moderate (638 mg) **
    Exchanges: 1¼ Meat, 2½ Bread, 1¼ Veg, 2¼ Fat

CAPELLINI CON POMODORO E BASILICO - SPECIAL REQUEST
Angel hair pasta, fresh tomato, fresh garlic and fresh basil. Request less oil (1 Tbs).
- ✓ CALORIES: Low (496)   ✓✓ CHOLESTEROL: None (0 mg)
- ✓ FAT: Low* (16 g)   ✓✓ SODIUM: Very Low (19 mg) **
    Exchanges: 4¼ Bread, 2 Veg, 2¾ Fat

SPIEDINI DI SCAMPI ALLE VERDURE
Skewers of shrimps and vegetables. Rice and polenta not included in analysis.
- ✓ CALORIES: Low (428)   CHOLESTEROL: High (380 mg)
- ✓ FAT: Low* (17 g)   ✓ SODIUM: Low (552 mg) **
    Exchanges: 4½ Meat (extra lean), 2¾ Veg, 2¾ Fat

PAILLARD DI POLLO
Grilled breast of chicken marinated in fresh herbs & extra virgin olive oil and served with steamed vegetables.
- ✓ CALORIES: Low (467)   CHOLESTEROL: Moderate (173 mg)
- ✓ FAT: Low (17 g)   ✓✓ SODIUM: Very Low (224 mg) **
    Exchanges: 9 Meat (extra lean), 2¼ Veg, 1¾ Fat

FRESH FISH PALERMITANA - SPECIAL REQUEST
Request less oil (½ oz). Analysis is for red snapper and steamed vegetables.
- ✓ CALORIES: Low (409)   ✓ CHOLESTEROL: Low (83 mg)
- ✓ FAT: Low* (17 g)   ✓✓ SODIUM: Very Low (278 mg) **
    Exchanges: 4¼ Meat (extra lean), 2½ Veg, 2¾ Fat

SCOTT'S
SEAFOOD
GRILL & BAR
Serving Finest Seafood
& Prime Steaks

Scott's reputation for serving the freshest seafood, classically prepared, in warm, relaxed and inviting surroundings has taken the tradition of quality and service to new heights. With its striking architecture, reminiscent of a gracious plantation home, Scott's Seafood has quickly become one of Orange County's landmark locations. The talented chefs create deceptively simple dishes that enhance the natural flavors of the freshest seafood available. Scott's Seafood ensures that each dining experience is a memorable one. $$

Scott's Seafood Grill and Bar
South Coast Plaza Town Center
3300 Bristol St., Costa Mesa, CA 92626   (714) 979-2400

SCOTT'S SEAFOOD SALAD - SPECIAL REQUEST
Poached scallops, dungeness crabmeat and bay shrimp on a bed of mixed lettuce with egg, tomato and cucumber. Request dressing on the side (not included in analysis).
- ✓✓ CALORIES: Very Low (236)
- CHOLESTEROL: Moderate (227 mg)
- ✓✓ FAT: Very Low (7 g)
- ✓ SODIUM: Low (532 mg) **
- Exchanges: 2½ Meat (extra lean), 2 Veg, ¾ Fat

FETTUCCINE FRUTTI DI MARE - SPECIAL REQUEST
with fresh fish, calamari, clams, mussels, prawns, tomatoes, peppers, olive oil, garlic and basil. Request less oil (½ oz).
- ✓ CALORIES: Low (595)
- CHOLESTEROL: (305 mg)
- ✓ FAT: Low* (20 g)
- ✓✓ SODIUM: Very Low (238 mg) **
- Exchanges: 3¼ Meat (extra lean), 3 Bread, 1 Veg, 3½ Fat

BLACKENED FILLET OF HAWAIIAN MAHI MAHI - SPECIAL REQUEST
with roasted garlic mashed potatoes and vegetables. Request less butter (1 tsp) and chutney sauce on the side (not included in analysis).
- ✓ CALORIES: Low (448)
- CHOLESTEROL: Moderate (186 mg)
- ✓ FAT: Low (19 g)
- SODIUM: Moderate (723 mg) **
- Exchanges: 3 Meat (extra lean), 1¼ Bread, 2 Veg, 3½ Fat

CHARBROILED FILLET OF PACIFIC SWORDFISH - SPECIAL REQUEST
with roasted tomato vinaigrette and carrot puree. Request vinaigrette prepared with less oil (1 tsp). Rice pilaf not included in analysis.
- ✓ CALORIES: Low (477)
- ✓ CHOLESTEROL: Low (92 mg)
- ✓ FAT: Low (20 g)
- ✓ SODIUM: Low (376 mg) **
- Exchanges: 4½ Meat, 1¼ Bread, 1¾ Veg, 2½ Fat

* Primarily unsaturated fat
** If you request no added salt

Sizzler®

Sizzler is famous for affordable, delicious and comfortable family dining. Our grill menu features fresh, lean steaks that are hand cut daily, and boneless skinless breast of chicken that is marinated and grilled to perfection. Our salad bar offers even more variety. From fresh fruit, crisp vegetables and tasty salads to pasta with marinara sauce and hot, steaming soups, our salad bar offers an endless variety of delicious, healthy items that you can select to suit your tastes and nutritional needs. At Sizzler, delicious healthy dining sounds good. $

Sizzler with 27 Orange County locations

LEMON-HERB CHICKEN
Tender 8 oz chicken breast seasoned in lemon and herbs.

✓✓ CALORIES: Very Low (213)   ✓ CHOLESTEROL: Low (134 mg)
✓✓ FAT: Very Low (5 g)   SODIUM: Moderate (837 mg)

TROUT - SPECIAL REQUEST
Request prepared without buttery oil.

✓✓ CALORIES: Very Low (221)   ✓ CHOLESTEROL: Low (97 mg)
✓✓ FAT: Very Low (8 g)   ✓✓ SODIUM: Very Low (91 mg)

HIBACHI CHICKEN BREAST
A savory 8 oz chicken breast broiled and basted with Hibachi sauce.

✓✓ CALORIES: Very Low (234)   ✓ CHOLESTEROL: Low (134 mg)
✓✓ FAT: Very Low (5 g)   SODIUM: High (1027 mg)

SHRIMP & SCALLOP SKEWERS
Three delicious shrimp and scallop skewers delicately seasoned with herbs.

✓✓ CALORIES: Very Low (220)   CHOLESTEROL: Moderate (160 mg)
✓✓ FAT: Very Low* (8 g)   SODIUM: Moderate (765 mg)

SIZZLER'S FAMOUS SOUP AND SALAD BAR *(selections may vary)*

✓✓ Very Low		✓ Low
(Under 20 calories and 1 g fat per ¼ cup)		*(Under 70 calories & 2 g fat per ¼ cup)*
Alfalfa Sprouts	Lemon wedges	Croutons
Broccoli	Beets	Garbanzo Beans
Cucumbers	Jicama	Salsa
Sliced Onion	Lettuce	Kidney Beans
Mushrooms	Red cabbage	Pasta (plain)
Tomatoes	Zucchini	Cottage Cheese (low-fat)
Spinach	Red & green peppers	Chicken Vegetable Soup
Seasonal Fresh Fruit		Vegetarian Vegetable Soup

Recommended Toppings: Low-cal Italian dressing, Low-cal French dressing, Salsa

† Side dish guidelines are 1/3 of entree guidelines
✓ Low   ✓✓ Very Low

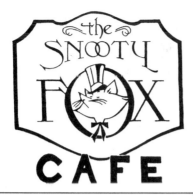

Snooty Fox Cafe... hearty down-home cooking, casual atmosphere, and country-club service. Breakfast, lunch and dinner served all day. $

Snooty Fox Cafe

30242 Crown Valley Parkway
Laguna Niguel, CA 92677
(714) 495-2298

CRANBERRY CHICKEN
Chicken breast with cranberry maple glaze and cranberry chutney.
✓ CALORIES: Low (595)   ✓ CHOLESTEROL: Low (130 mg)
✓✓ FAT: Very Low (10 g)   ✓✓ SODIUM: Very Low (152 mg) **
Exchanges: 6¾ Meat (extra lean), 4½ Fruit, 1 Fat

FRUIT AND COTTAGE CHEESE SALAD
*Fruit, cottage cheese, and mixed fresh greens. We recommend
low-fat dressing (not included in analysis).*
✓✓ CALORIES: Very Low (347)   ✓✓ CHOLESTEROL: Very Low (25 mg)
✓✓ FAT: Very Low (9 g)   SODIUM: Moderate (711 mg) **
Exchanges: 3 Meat, ½ Veg, 2¾ Fruit

BAKED FISH WITH TOMATOES AND MUSHROOMS
in white wine & herb sauce. Analysis is for red snapper; other fish similar.
✓✓ CALORIES: Very Low (336)   ✓ CHOLESTEROL: Low (94 mg)
✓✓ FAT: Very Low* (9 g)   ✓✓ SODIUM: Very Low (226 mg) **
Exchanges: 4¾ Meat (extra lean), 1 Veg, 1 Fat

VEGGIE PENNE - SPECIAL REQUEST
with mushrooms and simmered vegetables. Request no butter.
✓ CALORIES: Low (529)   ✓✓ CHOLESTEROL: None (0 mg)
✓✓ FAT: Very Low (3 g)   SODIUM: High (1232 mg)
Exchanges: 5¼ Bread, 4¼ Veg, ¼ Fat

DESSERT: BAKED APPLE†
CALORIES: Moderate (421)   ✓✓ CHOLESTEROL: Very Low (5 mg)
✓✓ FAT: Very Low (3 g)   ✓✓ SODIUM: Very Low (45 mg) **
Exchanges: 5 Fruit, ½ Fat

RECOMMENDED SIDE DISHES:
Rice Pilaf, Baked Potato (plain), Fresh Fruit, Steamed Vegetables,
French Bread (request no butter), or Salad with low-fat dressing.

---

* Primarily unsaturated fat
** If you request no added salt

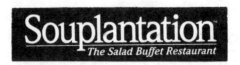

As one of the original salad buffet restaurants, Souplantation has maintained freshness as a way of life since 1978. We serve only the finest greens and produce and never use fresheners. All of our salad dressings are made from our own original recipes. All our soups and chilies are made from scratch each day, and our made-from-scratch muffins and breads are served warm from the oven. $

Souplantation Locations:

Brea: 555 Pointe Dr. Bldg 2   990-4773   Garden Grove: 5939 W. Chapman Ave. 895-1314
Costa Mesa: 1555 Adams Ave. 556-1903   Laguna Niguel: 23870 Aliso Creek Rd. 831-6055
Fountain Valley: 11179 Talbert 434-1814   Tustin: 13681 Newport Avenue   730-5443

LOW-FAT MUFFINS†
APPLE CINNAMON BRAN, CRANBERRY ORANGE BRAN, OR FRUIT MEDLEY BRAN
96% fat-free, made from scratch, and served warm from the oven. Analysis for 1 muffin.
- ✓✓ CALORIES: Very Low (80)
- ✓✓ FAT: Very Low* (½ g)
- ✓✓ CHOLESTEROL: None (0 mg)
- ✓ SODIUM: Low (110 mg)

LOW-FAT SOUPS & CHILIES†
Chicken Tortilla Soup, Classic Chicken Noodle Soup, Santa Fe Black Bean Chili, Sweet Tomato Onion Soup, Turkey Noodle Soup, or Vegetable Medley Soup. 1 cup serving contains:
- ✓ CALORIES: Low (90 to 190)
- ✓✓ FAT: Very Low (1 to 3 g)
- ✓✓ CHOLESTEROL: Very Low (0 to 30 mg)
- SODIUM: High (450 to 900 mg)

FAT-FREE PREPARED SALADS†
Red Pepper Slaw, Cucumber Tomato with Chile Lime Vinaigrette, Marinated Summer Vegetables. ½ cup contains:
- ✓✓ CALORIES: Very Low (20 to 80)
- ✓✓ FAT: None (0 g)
- ✓✓ CHOLESTEROL: None (0 mg)
- SODIUM: Cucumber...with Vinaigrette 20 mg; others 210 to 480 mg

LOW-FAT PREPARED SALADS†
Baja Bean & Cilantro, Carrot Raisin, Gemelli Pasta with Chicken in Citrus Vinaigrette, German Potato, Mandarin Krab, Mandarin Noodles with Broccoli, Mandarin Shells with Almonds, Mediterranean Harvest, Moroccan Marinated Vegetables, Oriental Ginger Slaw with Krab, Southern Dill Potato, Spicy Southwestern Pasta, Summer Barley with Black Beans. ½ cup contains:
- ✓ CALORIES: Low (70 to 180)
- ✓✓ FAT: Very Low* (3 g)
- ✓✓ CHOLESTEROL: Very Low (0 to 5 mg)
- SODIUM: Carrot Raisin 80 mg; Oriental Ginger 80 mg; others 180 to 380 mg

HOT PASTA WITH SAUCE†
1 cup plain or spinach pasta with ½ cup Italian Bruschetta fat-free sauce. Marinara is higher in calories & sodium.
- CALORIES: Moderate (390)
- ✓✓ FAT: Very Low* (3 g)
- ✓✓ CHOLESTEROL: None (0 mg)
- SODIUM: High (430 mg)

DESSERTS†
Chocolate, Tapioca, Vanilla or Rice Pudding, Nutty Waldorf Salad, Vanilla Soft Serve (½ cup) or small Cookie.
- ✓ CALORIES: Low (70 to 140)
- ✓✓ FAT: Very Low to Low (3 to 4 g)
- ✓✓ CHOLESTEROL: Very Low (0 to 20 mg)
- SODIUM: Rice Pudding, Soft Serve, Waldorf Salad & Cookie 50 to 80 mg; others 160 to 220 mg

Nutrition information supplied by Souplantation.

† Side dish guidelines are 1/3 of entree guidelines
✓ Low ✓✓ Very Low

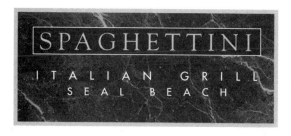

Spaghettini, a Northern Italian inspired grill, offers a variety of homemade pasta, pizza, fresh fish, meats and fowl. To complement your meal, Spaghettini offers an extensive wine list featuring both California and Italian wines (many available by the glass). The full cocktail lounge offers one of the largest back bars in Southern California with Happy Hour Monday through Friday 4-7 pm. Six nights of the week (Tuesday through Sunday), Spaghettini showcases live jazz, featuring top name groups, as well as up and coming talent, ranging from traditional to contemporary styles. Conveniently located at the 405 Freeway & Seal Beach Blvd. $$

Spaghettini Italian Grill

3005 Old Ranch Parkway, Seal Beach, CA 90740   (310) 596-2199

GRILLED NEW ZEALAND LAMB CHOP SALAD - SPECIAL REQUEST

A salad of mixed baby greens tossed with balsamic vinaigrette, roasted bell peppers and goat cheese, then topped with grilled lamb chops. Request less cheese (1 oz) and dressing on the side (dressing not included in analysis).

✓ CALORIES: Low (383)   ✓ CHOLESTEROL: Low (126 mg)
✓ FAT: Low (20 g)   ✓✓ SODIUM: Very Low (196 mg) **
Exchanges: 5½ Meat, 1¼ Veg, 1¼ Fat

LINGUINE WITH CLAMS - SPECIAL REQUEST

Homemade linguini tossed with our own clam sauce and steamed clams. Request less butter (½ oz).

✓ CALORIES: Low (541)   ✓ CHOLESTEROL: Low (118 mg)
✓ FAT: Low (15 g)   ✓ SODIUM: Low (578 mg) **
Exchanges: 2 Meat (extra lean), 4¼ Bread, 1 Veg, 2½ Fat

ANGEL HAIR PASTA AL FRESCA - SPECIAL REQUEST

Angel hair pasta tossed with Roma tomatoes, sweet basil and garlic. Request less oil (½ oz).

✓ CALORIES: Low (496)   ✓✓ CHOLESTEROL: Very Low (53 mg)
✓ FAT: Low* (16 g)   ✓✓ SODIUM: Very Low (28 mg) **
Exchanges: 4¼ Bread, ¼ Meat, 1¾ Veg, 2¾ Fat

CIOPPINO DEL MARE

A larger terrine of our cioppino style soup brimming with shrimp, grilled fresh fish and fresh seasonal shellfish over red pepper risotto. Served with garlic bread (not included in analysis).

✓ CALORIES: Low (419)   CHOLESTEROL: Moderate (263 mg)
✓✓ FAT: Very Low* (8 g)   SODIUM: Moderate (904 mg) **
Exchanges: 5½ Meat (extra lean), 1½ Bread, ½ Veg

* Primarily unsaturated fat
** If you request no added salt

The Sports Club/Irvine Bar and Grill is one of Irvine's best kept secrets, offering a fun, lively bistro atmosphere. We feature Euro-California cuisine, with special attention given to the epicurean "health palette" of our times. Open weekdays from 11:30 am - 3:00 pm and 5:00 pm to 9:00 pm. $

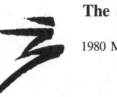

The Sports Club/Irvine Bar & Grill
1980 Main St, Irvine, CA 92714
(714) 975-8400

THE SPORTS CLUB/IRVINE

HEAVEN CAN WAIT
Angel hair tossed with mixed seasonal vegetables, mushrooms, tomatoes, garlic, basil & olive oil.

✓ CALORIES: Low (448)   ✓✓ CHOLESTEROL: None (0 mg)
✓ FAT: Low (15 g)   ✓✓ SODIUM: Very Low (8 mg) **
Exchanges: 4 Bread, 1¼ Veg, 2¾ Fat

PLYMOUTH ROCK SANDWICH
Chargrilled 6 oz turkey burger, lettuce, tomato, Bermuda onions and non-fat 1000 Island dressing on a toasted bun. Served with fresh fruit or non-fat BBQ potato salad (analyses below).

✓ CALORIES: Low (561)   ✓✓ CHOLESTEROL: Very Low (69 mg)
✓ FAT: Low (20 g)   SODIUM: Moderate (691 mg) **
Exchanges: 3¾ Meat, 3¾ Bread, ½ Veg, 1¾ Fat

RUE DE PARIS SANDWICH - SPECIAL REQUEST
Chargrilled double breast of chicken with lettuce, tomato, avocado and Dijon fat-free mayo on a toasted baguette. Served with fresh fruit or non-fat BBQ potato salad (analyses below). <u>Request no cheese.</u>

CALORIES: Moderate (703)   ✓ CHOLESTEROL: Low (130 mg)
✓ FAT: Low (13 g)   SODIUM: High (1360 mg)
Exchanges: 6¾ Meat (extra lean), 5½ Bread, ¼ Veg, 1 Fat

LEAN AND MEAN
Chargrilled double breast of chicken, with baked potato and steamed vegetables.

✓ CALORIES: Low (600)   ✓ CHOLESTEROL: Low (130 mg)
✓✓ FAT: Very Low (6 g)   ✓✓ SODIUM: Very Low (143 mg) **
Exchanges: 6¾ Meat (extra lean), 4 Bread, 1½ Veg

FISHERMAN'S WHARF - SPECIAL REQUEST
Fresh fish with vegetables, beans and rice pilaf (analysis for rice pilaf below). <u>Request less olive oil (½ Tbs) & vegetables steamed.</u> Analysis is for halibut; other fish similar.

✓ CALORIES: Low (551)   ✓✓ CHOLESTEROL: Very Low (73 mg)
✓ FAT: Low* (13 g)   ✓✓ SODIUM: Very Low (128 mg) **
Exchanges: 4½ Meat (extra lean), 2½ Bread, ¾ Veg, 1¼ Fat

FRESH FRUIT *(3 oz)*: 30 calories; <½ g fat; 0 cholesterol; 8 mg sodium**; Exch: ½ Fruit
NON-FAT BBQ POTATO SALAD *(4 oz)*: 66 calories; <½ g fat; 0 cholesterol; 460 mg sodium**; Exch: 1 Bread
RICE PILAF *(6 oz)*: 246 calories; 3 g fat; 56 mg cholesterol; 305 mg sodium**; Exch: 3 Bread, ½ Fat

✓ Low   ✓✓ Very Low

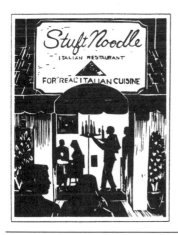

The Stuft Noodle is one of the locals' favorite restaurants. Serving gold award winning Italian cuisine, the Stuft Noodle also has an outstanding wine list and full bar, as well as banquet facilities and complete catering service.

The items shown here are specially designed and prepared for Healthy Dining, and must be ordered from the Healthy Dining menu. However we can also make any dish on our menu in non-stick pans without any oil or salt if requested. $$

The Stuft Noodle
215 Riverside Ave., Newport Beach, CA 92663   (714) 646-2333

CAPELLINI POLLO PRIMAVERA - SPECIAL REQUEST
Request "Healthy Dining Preparation."
CALORIES: Moderate (602)   ✓ CHOLESTEROL: Low (108 mg)
✓ FAT: Low (12 g)   ✓✓ SODIUM: Very Low (189 mg) **
Exchanges: 5¾ Meat (extra lean), 3 Bread, 3¾ Veg, 1 Fat

FETTUCINE WITH SHRIMP & SCALLOPS - SPECIAL REQUEST
Request "Healthy Dining Preparation."
CALORIES: Moderate (636)   CHOLESTEROL: Moderate (223 mg)
✓✓ FAT: Very Low* (5 g)   ✓ SODIUM: Low (516 mg) **
Exchanges: 3½ Meat (extra lean), 5½ Bread, ¾ Veg, ¼ Fat

GRILLED SWORDFISH CALABRESE - SPECIAL REQUEST
Request "Healthy Dining Preparation."
✓ CALORIES: Low (471)   ✓✓ CHOLESTEROL: Very Low (73 mg)
✓ FAT: Low* (13 g)   ✓✓ SODIUM: Very Low (153 mg) **
Exchanges: 4½ Meat (extra lean), 1½ Bread, 1 Veg, ¼ Fruit, 1½ Fat

POLLO BALTINO - SPECIAL REQUEST
Breast of chicken with artichoke hearts, mushrooms and tomato sauce.
Request "Healthy Dining Preparation."
✓ CALORIES: Low (546)   CHOLESTEROL: Moderate (173 mg)
✓✓ FAT: Very Low (10 g)   ✓ SODIUM: Low (301 mg) **
Exchanges: 9 Meat (extra lean), 1½ Bread, 3 Veg, ¼ Fat

FRESH FISH PALLARDE - SPECIAL REQUEST
Request "Healthy Dining Preparation."
✓ CALORIES: Low (403)   ✓✓ CHOLESTEROL: Very Low (73 mg)
✓✓ FAT: Very Low* (6 g)   ✓✓ SODIUM: Very Low (151 mg) **
Exchanges: 4½ Meat (extra lean), 1½ Bread, 1 Veg

EGGPLANT PARMIGIANA - SPECIAL REQUEST
Request "Healthy Dining Preparation."
✓✓ CALORIES: Very Low (292)   ✓✓ CHOLESTEROL: Very Low (22 mg)
✓✓ FAT: Very Low (8 g)   ✓✓ SODIUM: Very Low (205 mg) **
Exchanges: ¾ Meat, 2¼ Bread, 1¼ Veg, 1 Fat

---

* Primarily unsaturated fat
** If you request no added salt

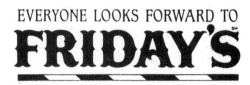

EVERYONE LOOKS FORWARD TO

Good Times & Great Food

Friday's® has an international reputation for its trend-setting menu and innovative foods, along with its dedication to providing flawless guest service in a fun atmosphere. The menu currently features a wide variety of over 90 food items, combining exotic fare with all-American favorites. Come and experience why Everyone Looks Forward to Friday's®! $

T.G.I. Friday's®

Brea - 935 E. Birch Street, Brea, CA 92621 (714) 256-2390
Costa Mesa - 601 Anton Blvd., Costa Mesa, CA 92626 (714) 540-2227
Laguna Niguel - 28141 Crown Valley Pkwy, Laguna Niguel, CA 92677 (714) 362-9770
Orange - 3339 City Parkway E, Orange, CA 92668 (714) 978-3308

PACIFIC COAST TUNA
A medley of steamed fresh seasonal vegetables with slices of charbroiled tuna steak atop linguini. Served with fat-free plum sauce# or oriental vinaigrette# for dipping.
   ✓ CALORIES: Low (410)   ✓✓ CHOLESTEROL: Very Low (70 mg)
  ✓✓ FAT: Very Low (7½ g)

PACIFIC COAST CHICKEN
A medley of steamed fresh seasonal vegetables with slices of charbroiled chicken breast atop linguini. Served with fat-free plum sauce# or oriental vinaigrette# for dipping.
   ✓ CALORIES: Low (415)   ✓✓ CHOLESTEROL: Very Low (70 mg)
  ✓✓ FAT: Very Low (8 g)

FRIDAY'S GARDENBURGER
The original gardenburger® made with whole grains, cheeses & mushrooms, on a whole wheat kaiser roll with lettuce, onion, tomato, pickle, chili yogurt sauce#, and black-eyed pea & corn salsa#.
   ✓ CALORIES: Low (445)   ✓✓ CHOLESTEROL: Very Low (13 mg)
  ✓✓ FAT: Very Low (9 g)

FRESH VEGETABLE MEDLEY
Fresh zucchini, squash, cauliflower, peppers, broccoli, carrots, snow peas and mushrooms, steamed and served with choice of brown rice pilaf or baked potato topped with low-fat Swiss cheese. Served with fat-free plum sauce# or oriental vinaigrette# for dipping and a House Salad. Analysis includes potato (rice slightly lower in calories and cholesterol).
   ✓ CALORIES: Low (470)   ✓✓ CHOLESTEROL: Very Low (25 mg)
  ✓✓ FAT: Very Low (8 g)

SALAD AND BAKED POTATO
Our House Salad offered with your choice of fat-free dressing.
Served alongside a baked potato with our chili yogurt sauce# and green onions.
  ✓✓ CALORIES: Very Low (250)   ✓✓ CHOLESTEROL: Very Low (2 mg)
  ✓✓ FAT: Very Low (½ g)

BLACK-EYED PEA & CORN SALSA: 175 calories & 2½ g fat. CHILI YOGURT: 30 calories & 0 fat.
PLUM SAUCE: 105 calories & 0 fat. ORIENTAL VINAIGRETTE: 180 calories & 14 g fat.

Nutrition information supplied by T.G.I. Friday's®

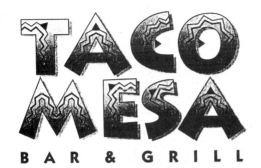

B A R & G R I L L

Taco Mesa offers authentic meals made from the finest ingredients. Lean cooking methods such as broiling, grilling and steaming assure that fresh foods stay that way. We do not cook with lard, MSG, preservatives, coloring or other additives. The Calderon family has been in the Mexican food business for 3 generations. We take pride in our commitment to quality, unique, authentic Mexican food at an affordable price. $

Taco Mesa   295 E. Imperial Highway, Fullerton, CA 92635   (714) 773-1273
647 West 19th Street, Costa Mesa, CA 92626   (714) 642-0629
22922 Los Alisos Blvd, Mission Viejo, CA 92691 (714) 472-3144

FRESH FRUIT SALAD (FULLERTON LOCATION ONLY)
Seasonal fresh fruit, coconut, assorted nuts and Taco Mesa sorbet.
Fresh fruit available at Costa Mesa and Mission Viejo locations.
✓✓ CALORIES: Very Low (344)   ✓✓ CHOLESTEROL: None (0 mg)
✓✓ FAT: Very Low* (4 g)   ✓✓ SODIUM: Very Low (55 mg) **
Exchanges: 3½ Fruit, ¼ Bread, ½ Fat

TACO DE SALMON - SPECIAL REQUEST
Fresh salmon on a flour tortilla with papaya sauce and papaya relish.
Request broiled and sauce on the side (sauce not included in analysis).
✓✓ CALORIES: Very Low (272)   ✓✓ CHOLESTEROL: Very Low (53 mg)
✓✓ FAT: Very Low* (9 g)   ✓✓ SODIUM: Very Low (213 mg) **
Exchanges: 2½ Meat, 1¼ Bread, ¼ Veg, ¼ Fruit, ½ Fat

BLACKENED FRESH FISH TACOS - SPECIAL REQUEST
Two tacos on flour tortillas with cabbage relish. Request no dairy (cheese, mayo, or sour cream).
✓✓ CALORIES: Very Low (306)   ✓✓ CHOLESTEROL: Very Low (35 mg)
✓ FAT: Low (12 g)   SODIUM: Moderate (866 mg) **
Exchanges: 1½ Meat (extra lean), 1¾ Bread, ¼ Veg, 2¼ Fat

GRILLED CHICKEN & PAPAYA SALAD - SPECIAL REQUEST
(FULLERTON LOCATION ONLY)
Mixed greens, chicken breast, papaya, onion, jicama, cucumber and other vegetables with achiote. Request cilantro dressing on the side (not included in analysis).
✓✓ CALORIES: Very Low (248)   ✓✓ CHOLESTEROL: Very Low (43 mg)
✓✓ FAT: Very Low (3 g)   ✓ SODIUM: Low (358 mg) **
Exchanges: 2¼ Meat (extra lean), 1¼ Veg, 2 Fruit

CHICKEN SKEWERS - SPECIAL REQUEST (FULLERTON LOCATION ONLY)
Served with rice and Mexican slaw with lemon butter sauce.
Request sauce on the side (slaw and sauce not included in analysis).
✓ CALORIES: Low (427)   ✓ CHOLESTEROL: Low (142 mg)
✓ FAT: Low (13 g)   SODIUM: Moderate (875 mg) **
Exchanges: 7½ Meat (extra lean), 1 Bread, ½ Veg, 1½ Fat

* Primarily unsaturated fat
** If you request no added salt

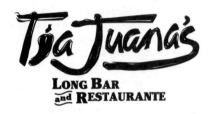

**LONG BAR
and RESTAURANTE**

You'll feel like you've been transported across the border at Tia Juana's, with brightly colored banners, our famous handshaken margaritas and authentic Mexican cuisine. Our salsas, sauces, and tortillas are made fresh daily by our cocineros (cooks). Tia Juana's also offers traditional American dishes, as well as banquet parties & meetings for 10-300. Live music Tues. - Sat., ranging from rock & roll to South American folk tunes. Sporting enthusiasts can also catch all the action on our 10-foot Panasonic Big Screen and 30-inch TV's. $

Tia Juana's 14988 Sand Canyon Avenue, Irvine, CA 92718 (714) 551-2998

VEGETABLE FAJITAS
A sizzling do-it-yourself platter of sweet bell peppers, onions, ripe tomatoes and salsa rojas, served with fresh handmade tortillas. Analysis includes 3 tortillas, but not sour cream or guacamole. Also served with Mexican rice and Tia Juana's refried beans (see analyses below).
✓ CALORIES: Low (552)   ✓✓ CHOLESTEROL: None (0 mg)
✓✓ FAT: Very Low* (10 g)   SODIUM: Moderate (996 mg) **
Exchanges: 4¾ Bread, 5¼ Veg, 1¾ Fat

TACOS SAN FELIPE - SPECIAL REQUEST
Handmade flour tortillas filled with sauteed sea bass, fresh pico de gallo and Tia Juana's blend of special spices. Request no cheese. Served with Mexican rice and Tia Juana's refried beans (analyses below). Corn cake not included in analysis.
✓ CALORIES: Low (510)   ✓✓ CHOLESTEROL: Very Low (47 mg)
✓ FAT: Low* (18 g)   SODIUM: Moderate (687 mg) **
Exchanges: 2 Meat, 3¼ Bread, ½ Veg, ¼ Fruit, 3 Fat

STEAMED VEGETABLE PLATE - SPECIAL REQUEST
Steamed chayote squash, broccoli, cauliflower, carrots and zucchini served on a bed of Mexican rice. Request cheese on the side (not included in analysis). Corn cake not included in analysis.
✓✓ CALORIES: Very Low (217)   ✓✓ CHOLESTEROL: None (0 mg)
✓✓ FAT: Very Low* (5 g)   ✓ SODIUM: Low (354 mg) **
Exchanges: 1¼ Bread, 3 Veg, ¾ Fat

TIA JUANA'S VEGGIE BURGER
Grilled, meatless, soy-free patty with the works! Served with fresh fruit. Corn cake not included in analysis.
✓ CALORIES: Low (577)   ✓✓ CHOLESTEROL: Very Low (8 mg)
✓✓ FAT: Very Low* (8 g)   SODIUM: High (1481 mg)
Exchanges: ½ Meat, 5¾ Bread, 1 Veg, ¾ Fruit, 1¼ Fat

TIA JUANA'S CHICKEN SALAD - SPECIAL REQUEST
Breast of chicken, mandarin oranges, green onions, celery, water chestnuts, almonds and sesame seeds. Served with a light honey-ginger-soy sauce marinade. Request less almonds & sesame seeds (1 Tbs. each) and dressing on the side (dressing not included in analysis).
✓ CALORIES: Low (489)   ✓ CHOLESTEROL: Low (108 mg)
✓ FAT: Low (15 g)   ✓ SODIUM: Low (360 mg) **
Exchanges: 5¾ Meat (extra lean), ½ Bread, 3¼ Veg, ¼ Fruit, 1 Fat

MEXICAN RICE *(4 oz)* 149 calories, 4 g fat, 0 cholesterol, 307 mg sodium
REFRIED BEANS - REQUEST NO CHEESE *(4 oz)* 194 calories, 6 g fat, 0 cholesterol, 219 mg sodium

The traditions of excellent Latin American food and charming surroundings continue to be observed with two delightful restaurants in Orange County -- the little old Laguna Charm "house" on Pacific Coast Highway and the Market-on-the-Lake overlooking Lake Mission Viejo. Tortilla Flats will welcome you and ask you to make yourself at home. Request "Healthy Dining Preparation" for items especially prepared with your health in mind. $$

Tortilla Flats

1740 S. Coast Hwy, Laguna Beach, CA 92651 (714) 494-6588
27792 Vista Del Lago, Mission Viejo, CA 92692 (714) 830-9980

POLLO PIBIL - SPECIAL REQUEST

A tender chicken breast baked in our delicious Yucatan achiote sauce flavored with the delicate taste of fresh oranges. Served with rice & beans (analyses below). Request "Healthy Dining Preparation."

✓ CALORIES: Low (363)   CHOLESTEROL: Moderate (173 mg)
✓✓ FAT: Very Low (7 g)   SODIUM: High (1271 mg)
Exchanges: 9 Meat (extra lean), ¼ Veg, ¼ Fruit

MARIPOSA Y CAMERONES - SPECIAL REQUEST

Butterflied breast of chicken charbroiled to juicy perfection, topped with sautéed pasilla chiles and onions, accompanied with succulent shrimp, smothered in spicy chile de arbol sauce. Served with rice (analysis below). Request "Healthy Dining Preparation."

✓ CALORIES: Low (509)   CHOLESTEROL: High (348 mg)
✓ FAT: Low (12 g)   SODIUM: Moderate (918 mg) **
Exchanges: 10¾ Meat (extra lean), 1 Veg, ¼ Fruit, ¾ Fat

ENCHILADA DE CANGREJO Y CAMERONES - SPECIAL REQUEST

Crab and shrimp enchilada with onions, avocado, cotija cheese, chile de arbol sauce & seasonings. Served with rice & beans (analyses below). Request "Healthy Dining Preparation."

✓ CALORIES: Low (403)   CHOLESTEROL: Moderate (299 mg)
✓ FAT: Low* (11 g)   SODIUM: High (1638 mg)
Exchanges: 4½ Meat (extra lean), ¾ Bread, 1 Veg, ¼ Veg, 1½ Fat

POLLO DON RAMON - SPECIAL REQUEST

Tender pieces of boned chicken breasts slightly sautéed with tomatoes, onions, chiles, garlic and flavored with cilantro. Served with rice (analysis below). Request "Healthy Dining Preparation."

✓ CALORIES: Low (412)   CHOLESTEROL: Moderate (173 mg)
✓✓ FAT: Very Low (8 g)   SODIUM: High (1016 mg)
Exchanges: 9 (extra lean), 2¾ Veg

PESCADO CON ROJAS - SPECIAL REQUEST

Charbroiled swordfish steak with sautéed pasilla chiles and onions. Includes 2 corn tortillas. Served with rice and beans (analyses below). Request "Healthy Dining Preparation."

✓ CALORIES: Low (466)   ✓ CHOLESTEROL: Low (101 mg)
✓ FAT: Low (12 g)   ✓ SODIUM: Low (312 mg) **
Exchanges: 5¾ Meat, 1½ Bread, 1¼ Veg, ¼ Fat

FISH TACOS (A LA CARTE) - SPECIAL REQUEST

Two corn tortillas with red snapper, cabbage, cheese & salsa. Request "Healthy Dining Preparation."

✓✓ CALORIES: Very Low (232)   ✓✓ CHOLESTEROL: Very Low (39 mg)
✓✓ FAT: Very Low (5 g)   ✓✓ SODIUM: Very Low (233 mg) **
Exchanges: 1¾ Meat, 1½ Bread, ¼ Veg, ½ Fat

BEANS *(1 cup)* 238 calories; 1 g fat; 0 cholesterol; 197 mg sodium**; Exch: ¾ Meat, 3 Bread, ¼ Veg
RICE *(1 cup)* 181 calories; 1 g fat; 59 mg cholesterol; 122 mg sodium**; Exch: 2½ Bread

* Primarily unsaturated fat
** If you request no added salt

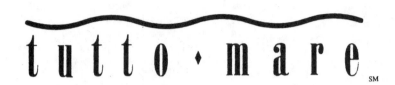

With over 3,000 miles of coastline, it's no surprise that Italy has delicious seafood dishes. Which is why Tutto Mare's award-winning menu is awash with specialties from Italy's seaside regions. Since seafood isn't the only thing Italians do well, we also serve homemade pastas, pizzas baked in an oak-fired oven, and meats prepared on the rotisserie. Come taste the cuisine that only the Mediterranean could inspire. $$

Tutto Mare

545 Newport Center Drive - Fashion Island, Newport Beach, CA 92660
(714) 640-6333

VERMICELLI AGLI SCAMPI

Thin spaghetti, langostino, baby clams, brandy & tomato sauce.
CALORIES: Moderate (689)   ✓ CHOLESTEROL: Low (95 mg)
✓✓ FAT: Very Low* (10 g)   ✓ SODIUM: Low (552 mg) **
Exchanges: 3 Meat (extra lean), 5½ Bread, 1 Veg, 1½ Fat

TAGLIOLINI CON GAMBERETTI E MELANZANE

Thin pasta, shrimp, eggplant, spicy tomato sauce and herbs.
✓ CALORIES: Low (600)   CHOLESTEROL: Moderate (249 mg)
✓ FAT: Low* (18 g)   ✓✓ SODIUM: Very Low (255 mg) **
Exchanges: 2½ Meat (extra lean), 3½ Bread, 1½ Veg, 2¾ Fat

GRIGLIATA MISTA DI PESCE

Mixed seafood grill of calamari, fresh fish and prawns.
✓ CALORIES: Low (430)   CHOLESTEROL: Moderate (314 mg)
✓ FAT: Low* (20 g)   ✓✓ SODIUM: Very Low (256 mg) **
Exchanges: 7½ Meat (extra lean), ¼ Fruit, 2¾ Fat

TAGLIERINI DEL FATTORE

Thin pasta with artichokes, leeks, spinach, lentils & tomato.
✓ CALORIES: Low (504)   ✓ CHOLESTEROL: Low (116 mg)
✓ FAT: Low* (19 g)   ✓✓ SODIUM: Very Low (188 mg) **
Exchanges: 4 Bread, 1¾ Veg, 3¾ Fat

STUFATO DI CANESTRELLI IN SALSA AROMATICA

Grilled scallops with sautéed mussels, white wine, arugula and steamed vegetables.
✓ CALORIES: Low (441)   ✓ CHOLESTEROL: Low (128 mg)
✓ FAT: Low (11 g)   SODIUM: Moderate (674 mg) **
Exchanges: 4¾ Meat (extra lean), 1¼ Bread, 1½ Veg, 1¼ Fat

New vegetarian food
from around the world
à GO-GO style!
Low in fat
Strong in flavor
Healthy not bland
and always fun!

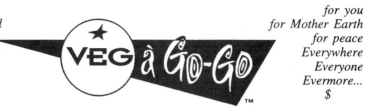

for you
for Mother Earth
for peace
Everywhere
Everyone
Evermore...
$

Veg à Go-Go
Atrium Court, Fashion Island, Newport Beach, CA 92660   (714) 721-4088

GO-GO BURGER OR MINI BURGERS
Meatless soy & cheese patty, with lettuce, tomato and our secret sauce on a light multi-grain bun. Analysis is for 1 Go-Go Burger; analysis for 2 Mini-Burgers is very similar.
✓✓ CALORIES: Very Low (244)   ✓✓ CHOLESTEROL: Very Low (3 mg)
✓✓ FAT: Very Low* (5 g)   ✓ SODIUM: Low (578 mg)
Exchanges: 1¾ Meat, 2 Bread, ½ Fat

RAPPERS: *More than a burrito - our special sandwiches rolled and wrapped in pita bread, low-fat flour or whole wheat tortilla.*

BBQ VEGGIES RAP
Lightly grilled broccoli, corn, carrots, onions, red & green peppers layered with natural barbeque sauce, "cheese" (fat-free soy cheese), & brown rice in a low-fat flour tortilla.
✓✓ CALORIES: Very Low (283)   ✓✓ CHOLESTEROL: None (0 mg)
✓✓ FAT: Very Low* (6 g)   SODIUM: High (1066 mg)
Exchanges: 1 Meat, 2¼ Bread, 2 Veg, 1 Fat

SPICY INDIAN RAPPER
Spicy Indian curry with chickpeas & stewed tomatoes, brown rice, lettuce and cabbage in a low-fat whole wheat tortilla.
✓✓ CALORIES: Very Low (269)   ✓✓ CHOLESTEROL: None (0 mg)
✓✓ FAT: Very Low* (6 g)   SODIUM: Moderate (716 mg)
Exchanges: 3 Bread, ½ Veg, ¾ Fat

FALAFELRAP
Our falafel, tahini dressing & salsa in pita with fresh lettuce & cabbage.
✓ CALORIES: Low (358)   ✓✓ CHOLESTEROL: None (0 mg)
✓✓ FAT: Very Low* (8 g)   SODIUM: High (1036 mg)
Exchanges: ½ Meat, 3½ Bread, ¾ Veg, 1¼ Fat

MOO SHU SHU RAPPER
Fresh bean sprouts, celery, spinach, carrots & cabbage, wok'd lightly and rolled in a low-fat flour tortilla, and our natural Hoisin sauce.
✓✓ CALORIES: Very Low (232)   ✓✓ CHOLESTEROL: None (0 mg)
✓✓ FAT: Very Low* (6 g)   SODIUM: Moderate (627 mg)
Exchanges: 1¼ Bread, 2¾ Veg, 1¼ Fat

THAI RAP
Spicy Thai vinaigrette, fresh cilantro, bean sprouts, carrots, broccoli & red cabbage in a low-fat tortilla.
✓✓ CALORIES: Very Low (248)   ✓✓ CHOLESTEROL: None (0 mg)
✓✓ FAT: Very Low* (9 g)   ✓ SODIUM: Low (407 mg)
Exchanges: ¼ Meat, 1¼ Bread, 1½ Veg, 1¾ Fat

SIDE DISH: AIR FRIES
Cooked in air and lightly seasoned with sea salt & spices.

---

* Primarily unsaturated fat
** If you request no added salt

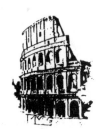

Villa Roma
Ristorante Italiano

Villa Roma -- "A trip to Italy without a passport!" We transport the tradition of authentic country food where everything is made with fresh ingredients. "That is the secret of a long and healthy life." The atmosphere is conducive to a relaxing, enjoyable dining experience, from the romantic lighting, crisp table linens and soft music lingering in the background to the attentive, eager-to-please staff. Live entertainment and dancing Wed-Sat. $

Villa Roma

23700-D El Toro Rd. (Saddleback Valley Plaza), Lake Forest, CA 92630 (714) 454-8585

CAPELLINI ALLA PRIMAVERA
Angel hair pasta with fresh tomato and fresh seasonal vegetables, tossed with garlic and olive oil with a touch of marinara sauce.
- ✓ CALORIES: Low (567)
- ✓ FAT: Low* (20 g)
- ✓✓ CHOLESTEROL: None (0 mg)
- ✓✓ SODIUM: Very Low (248 mg) **

Exchanges: 4¾ Bread, 2 Veg, 3½ Fat

PETTI DI POLLO ALLA GRIGLIA
Grilled chicken breast with rosemary sauce, served with pasta and marinara sauce.
- ✓ CALORIES: Low (545)
- ✓ FAT: Low (16 g)
- CHOLESTEROL: Moderate (173 mg)
- ✓✓ SODIUM: Very Low (229 mg) **

Exchanges: 9 Meat (extra lean), 1½ Bread, ¼ Veg, ¼ Fruit, 1½ Fat

SCAMPI VILLA ROMA
Jumbo shrimp with garlic, white wine, olive oil and lemon, served with pasta and marinara sauce.
- ✓ CALORIES: Low (414)
- ✓ FAT: Low* (17 g)
- CHOLESTEROL: Moderate (219 mg)
- ✓ SODIUM: Low (585 mg) **

Exchanges: 2 Meat (extra lean), 1½ Bread, ½ Veg, 3 Fat

CAPELLINI ALLA CHECCA
Angel hair pasta with fresh chopped tomato, garlic and fresh basil.
- ✓ CALORIES: Low (529)
- ✓ FAT: Low* (17 g)
- ✓✓ CHOLESTEROL: None (0 mg)
- ✓✓ SODIUM: Very Low (92 mg) **

Exchanges: 4¾ Bread, 1¼ Veg, 3 Fat

PESCE SPADA ALLA GRIGLIA
Grilled swordfish, tomato, herbs and wine, served with pasta and marinara sauce.
- ✓ CALORIES: Low (532)
- ✓ FAT: Low* (20 g)
- ✓ CHOLESTEROL: Low (89 mg)
- ✓ SODIUM: Low (584 mg) **

Exchanges: 5 Meat, 1½ Bread, 1 Veg, 2 Fat

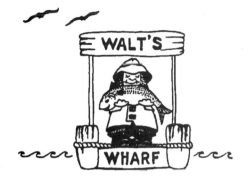

Located on Main Street in what Sunset Magazine describes as "The Last of America's Small Towns," Walt's Wharf offers the freshest seafood cooked over a red oak fire, lean Limousin beef, fresh homemade pastas and specially grown vegetables, all served in a comfortable, friendly neighborhood building built in the early 1930's. Walt Babcock, retired dentist and winery owner, has found a way to "take the guilt out of eating a juicy steak" by serving Limousin Beef from Nebraska. $$

Walt's Wharf   201 Main Street, Seal Beach, CA 90740   (310) 598-4433

HAWAIIAN BLACKENED AHI SALAD - SPECIAL REQUEST
Blackened ahi sashimi served with field greens, fresh papaya, roasted red peppers, wasabi aioli, roasted red pepper sauce and balsamic vinaigrette. Request dressing on the side (not included in analysis).

✓✓ CALORIES: Very Low (303) ✓✓ CHOLESTEROL: Very Low (60 mg)
✓✓ FAT: Very Low (10 g) ✓✓ SODIUM: Very Low (102 mg) **
Exchanges: 4¼ Meat (extra lean), 1 Bread, 1½ Veg, ¼ Fruit, 2 Fat

JALAPENO-LIME CHICKEN BREAST
with steamed vegetables and baked potato (request plain).

✓ CALORIES: Low (557) CHOLESTEROL: Moderate (162 mg)
✓ FAT: Low (12 g) ✓ SODIUM: Low (351 mg) **
Exchanges: 8½ Meat (extra lean), 2½ Bread, ½ Veg, 1 Fat

OAK GRILLED VEGETABLE PLATTER
Grilled artichoke, eggplant, bell pepper, zucchini, onion and squash served with lemon, garlic butter, and aioli (aioli not included in analysis).

✓✓ CALORIES: Very Low (270) ✓✓ CHOLESTEROL: Very Low (31 mg)
✓ FAT: Low (12 g) ✓✓ SODIUM: Very Low (262 mg) **
Exchanges: ¼ Bread, 5½ Veg, ¼ Fruit, 2¼ Fat

ORANGE ROUGHY WITH PAPAYA AND RED CHILE SALSA
with steamed vegetables and baked potato (request plain).

✓ CALORIES: Low (394) ✓✓ CHOLESTEROL: Very Low (45 mg)
✓✓ FAT: Very Low* (4 g) ✓✓ SODIUM: Very Low (163 mg) **
Exchanges: 2¾ Meat (extra lean), 2½ Bread, ¾ Veg, ¼ Fruit, ¼ Fat

OAK GRILLED LEAN LIMOUSIN FILET MIGNON
with Cabernet Sauvignon-enhanced demi-glacé, steamed vegetables, baked potato (request plain) and fried onions (not included in analysis).

✓ CALORIES: Low (456) ✓ CHOLESTEROL: Low (129 mg)
✓✓ FAT: Very Low (5 g) ✓ SODIUM: Low (342 mg) **
Exchanges: 6¾ Meat (extra lean), 2½ Bread, ½ Veg

---

* Primarily unsaturated fat
** If you request no added salt

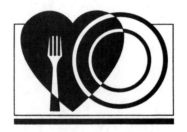

122   *Healthy Dining in Orange County*

Fast Food

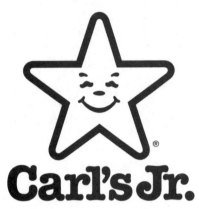

Carl's Jr.®

At Carl's Jr.®, we offer quality, nutrition and taste you can count on. Our Charbroiled BBQ Chicken Sandwich is big on taste but not on calories. Our Charbroiled Chicken Salad-To-Go™, Plain Potato and Garden Salad are all made of only the finest ingredients. At Carl's Jr., we offer fast food alternatives that make sensible nutrition part of a delicious meal. $

70 Orange County locations

CHARBROILED BBQ CHICKEN SANDWICH

✓✓ CALORIES: Very Low (310) ✓✓ CHOLESTEROL: Very Low (55 mg)
✓✓ FAT: Very Low (6 g) SODIUM: Moderate (830 mg)

CHARBROILED CHICKEN SALAD-TO-GO™

✓✓ CALORIES: Very Low (260) ✓✓ CHOLESTEROL: Very Low (70 mg)
✓✓ FAT: Very Low (9 g) ✓✓ SODIUM: Very Low (530 mg)

PLAIN POTATO

✓✓ CALORIES: Very Low (290) ✓✓ CHOLESTEROL: None (0 mg)
✓✓ FAT: None (0 g) ✓✓ SODIUM: Very Low (40 mg)

GARDEN SALAD†

✓✓ CALORIES: Very Low (50) ✓✓ CHOLESTEROL: Very Low (5 mg)
✓✓ FAT: Very Low (3 g) ✓✓ SODIUM: Very Low (75 mg)

Nutrition information supplied by Carl's Jr.®   ©1995 Carl Karcher Enterprises, Inc.

† Side dish guidelines are 1/3 of entree guidelines
✓ Low   ✓✓ Very Low

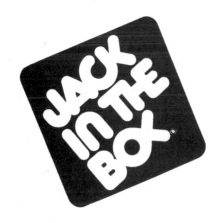

JACK IN THE BOX® prepares food that not only tastes great, but also provides the nutritional balance that people are looking for. We cook with only 100% cholesterol-free vegetable oil, a soybean/cottonseed blend that contains no tropical oils, and is low in saturated fat. And we're looking out for you with lowfat milk, farm fresh vegetables in our sandwiches and salads, and reduced calorie dressing. JACK IN THE BOX® has only one mission: to continually create the most exciting, best tasting fast food anywhere. $

CHICKEN TERIYAKI BOWL

Strips of teriyaki-marinated chicken breast, broccoli florets, carrots and teriyaki sauce, all served on a bed of steamed white rice.

✓ CALORIES: Low (580) ✓✓ CHOLESTEROL: Very Low (30 mg)
✓✓ FAT: Very Low (1½ g) SODIUM: High (1220 mg)
Exchanges: ½+ Meat, 6 Bread, 2½ Veg

CHICKEN FAJITA PITA

Tender chunks of all white meat chicken, natural cheddar cheese, tomatoes & lettuce. All in a pita pocket and all less than 300 calories. Guacamole and salsa not included in analysis.

✓✓ CALORIES: Very Low (290) ✓✓ CHOLESTEROL: Very Low (35 mg)
✓✓ FAT: Very Low (8 g) SODIUM: Moderate (700 mg)
Exchanges: 2 Meat, 2 Bread

GRILLED CHICKEN FILLET

Tender, boneless breast of chicken, lightly seasoned and grilled. Topped with cheese, tomatoes, lettuce and sauce on a toasted wheat bun.

✓ CALORIES: Low (430) ✓✓ CHOLESTEROL: Very Low (65 mg)
✓ FAT: Low (19 g) SODIUM: High (1070 mg)
Exchanges: 3 Meat, 2 Bread, 1 Fat

GARDEN CHICKEN SALAD

Iceberg & Romaine lettuce with strips of marinated chicken breast, natural cheddar cheese, fresh carrots and tomatoes. Dressing and croutons not included in analysis.

✓✓ CALORIES: Very Low (200) ✓✓ CHOLESTEROL: Very Low (65 mg)
✓✓ FAT: Very Low (9 g) ✓ SODIUM: Low (420 mg)
Exchanges: 3 Meat, 1 Veg, 1 Fat

Nutrition information supplied by JACK IN THE BOX®

* Primarily unsaturated fat

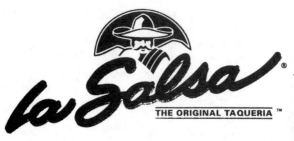

THE ORIGINAL TAQUERIA ™

Inspired by the famous street taquerias of Mexico City, La Salsa has grown to be Southern California's favorite family of Mexican restaurants. We serve only the freshest, healthiest gourmet food that is truly authentic. All of our meat is 95% fat-free and we use only canola or peanut oils. We make over 1 ton of fresh salsa daily and can accommodate most vegetarian requests. Customize your dish with the unique flavors found in our fresh salsa bar. Every La Salsa restaurant also features an enthusiastic staff that wants to share with you the wonderful Mexican tradition of food and hospitality. $

La Salsa locations:

Costa Mesa Triangle Square: 1870 Harbor Blvd, Costa Mesa, CA 92627   (714) 646-0397
Irvine Crossroads: 3850 Barranca Pkwy, Irvine, CA 92714   (714) 786-7692
Newport Beach Fashion Island: 401 Newport Ctr Dr, Newport Beach, CA   (714) 640-4289
South Coast -- Santa Ana: 3930 So. Bristol, Santa Ana, CA 92704   (714) 549-9974

Analysis does not include chips.

TACO LA SALSA - CHICKEN
Charbroiled chicken with cheese, salsa, lettuce, tomatoes and cilantro served on corn tortillas.
✓✓ CALORIES: Very Low (247)   ✓✓ CHOLESTEROL: Very Low (44 mg)
✓✓ FAT: Very Low (6 g)   ✓✓ SODIUM: Very Low (187 mg)
Exchanges: 2 Meat (extra lean), 1¾ Bread, ¼ Veg, ¾ Fat

MEXICO CITY TACO - CHICKEN
With charbroiled skinless chicken served on corn tortillas.
✓✓ CALORIES: Very Low (171)   ✓✓ CHOLESTEROL: Very Low (36 mg)
✓✓ FAT: Very Low (3 g)   ✓✓ SODIUM: Very Low (110 mg)
Exchanges: 1¾ Meat (extra lean), 1½ Bread, ¼ Fat

FISH TACO (SONORA STYLE)
Broiled mahi-mahi with cheese, lettuce, cilantro, and Salsa Sonora on a flour tortilla.
✓✓ CALORIES: Very Low (193)   ✓✓ CHOLESTEROL: Very Low (38 mg)
✓✓ FAT: Very Low (8 g)   ✓✓ SODIUM: Very Low (300 mg)
Exchanges: 1 Meat, 1¼ Bread, ¼ Veg, ¼ Fruit, 1¼ Fat

VEGETARIAN TACO
Our famous vegetarian black beans, cheese, avocado, grilled tomatoes & onions on corn tortillas.
✓✓ CALORIES: Very Low (280)   ✓✓ CHOLESTEROL: Very Low (7 mg)
✓✓ FAT: Very Low (7 g)   ✓✓ SODIUM: Very Low (159 mg)
Exchanges: ¼ Meat, 2½ Bread, ½ Veg, 1¼ Fat

BEAN AND CHEESE BURRITO
Our famous black beans and cheese.
✓ CALORIES: Low (560)   ✓✓ CHOLESTEROL: Very Low (30 mg)
✓ FAT: Low (16 g)   SODIUM: Moderate (750 mg)
Exchanges: 1 Meat, 5¼ Bread, 2½ Fat

BLACK BEANS AND RICE†
CALORIES: Moderate (273)   ✓✓ CHOLESTEROL: None (0 mg)
✓✓ FAT: Very Low* (3 g)   ✓✓ SODIUM: Very Low (60 mg)
Exchanges: 3 Bread, ½ Veg, ½ Fat

† Side dish guidelines are 1/3 of entree guidelines

   ✓ Low   ✓✓ Very Low

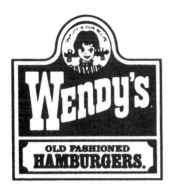

When Dave Thomas opened the first Wendy's Old Fashioned Hamburgers restaurant in 1969, his philosophy was simple: to serve fresh, high-quality food just like food made at home. Wendy's was the first hamburger chain to offer wholesome chili (1969), launch fresh salad bars nationwide (1979), offer a breast of chicken sandwich cooked in cholesterol-free vegetable oil (1981), and baked potatoes (1983). In 1990, Wendy's began cooking French fries in 100% corn oil and introduced the lower-fat Grilled Chicken Breast Fillet sandwich. Today Wendy's continues to provide a wide variety of quality choices, including those shown below. $

Wendy's Locations:
1150 Baker Street, Costa Mesa
468 E. 17th Street, Costa Mesa
17940 Brookhurst Ave, Fountain Valley
10040 Chapman Ave, Garden Grove
26792 Portola Parkway, Foothill Ranch
16082 Golden West Ave, Huntington Beach
14386 Culver Drive, Irvine

24761 Alicia Parkway, Laguna Hills
28961 Golden Lantern, Laguna Niguel
23572 El Toro Road, Lake Forest
1237 N. Tustin Ave, Orange
2640 S. Bristol Street, Santa Ana
1737 E. 17th Street, Santa Ana
12975 Beach Blvd, Stanton
2055 Westminster Mall, Westminster

CHILI (8 OZ) *with 2 saltine crackers*
✓✓ CALORIES: Very Low (235) ✓✓ CHOLESTEROL: Very Low (30 mg)
✓✓ FAT: Very Low (7 g) SODIUM: Moderate (880 mg)

GRILLED CHICKEN SANDWICH
Breast fillet with honey mustard sauce, tomato and lettuce.
✓✓ CALORIES: Very Low (290) ✓✓ CHOLESTEROL: Very Low (55 mg)
✓✓ FAT: Very Low (7 g) SODIUM: Moderate (720 mg)

BROCCOLI AND CHEESE STUFFED BAKED POTATO
✓ CALORIES: Low (470) ✓✓ CHOLESTEROL: Very Low (5 mg)
✓ FAT: Low (14 g) ✓ SODIUM: Low (470 mg)

GARDEN SPOT™ SALAD BAR CHOICES
✓✓ Very Low *The following recommended choices have less than 60 calories, less than 2 grams of fat, and less than 60 mg sodium per ¼ cup serving:*

Broccoli	Chives	Honeydew Melon	Bananas & Strawberry Glaze	
Cantaloupe	Cucumbers	Lettuce	Peaches	Strawberries
Carrots	Green Peas	Mushrooms	Pineapple	Tomatoes
Cauliflower	Green Peppers	Oranges	Red Onions	Watermelon

The following items should be eaten in only small quantities:

Bacon Bits	Cottage Cheese	Pasta Salad	Sunflower Seeds
Cheese	Croutons	Potato Salad	Tuna Salad
Chicken Salad	Egg	Seafood Salad	Turkey Ham
Cole Slaw	Olives, black	Pudding	Chow Mein Noodles

Nutrition information supplied by Wendy's.

* Primarily unsaturated fat

Markets, Delis
and Bakery

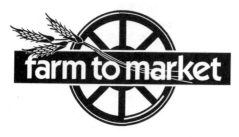

Farm to Market offers a complete selection of fresh-made entrees, salads, breads, rolls and pastries. All of our meals are prepared from scratch, using only the finest of ingredients -- just like you would use at home. We now offer a wide range of our more popular recipes in a low-fat or fat-free version. Experience our friendly, neighborhood service. $

Farm to Market

30190 Town Center Drive, Laguna Niguel, CA 92677   (714) 363-0123
23166 Los Alisos Blvd., Mission Viejo, CA 92691   (714) 458-0123
32382 Del Obispo St., San Juan Capistrano, CA 92675   (714) 493-0005

LOW-FAT STUFFED JUMBO SHELLS

with fat-free cheeses in a savory marinara sauce. Large (approx. 16 oz) serving.

✓ CALORIES: Low (355)   ✓✓ CHOLESTEROL: None (0 mg)
✓✓ FAT: Very Low (1 g)   SODIUM: Moderate (838 mg)
Exchanges: 2 Meat (extra lean), 2¼ Bread, 2½ Veg, ¾ Milk

TURKEY CHILI

A zesty homemade Texas-style chili with fresh ground skinless turkey instead of beef. All the taste but less fat! Large (approx. 16 oz) serving.

✓✓ CALORIES: Very Low (251)   ✓✓ CHOLESTEROL: Very Low (20 mg)
✓✓ FAT: Very Low (6 g)   SODIUM: Moderate (747 mg)
Exchanges: 1 Meat, 1¼ Bread, 2¼ Veg, ½ Fat

LINGUINI AND CLAM SAUCE

A light and flavorful clam sauce served over a bed of linguine that will satisfy your palate without that heavy feeling. Large (approx. 16 oz) serving.

✓ CALORIES: Low (382)   ✓✓ CHOLESTEROL: Very Low (16 mg)
✓✓ FAT: Very Low* (3 g)   ✓ SODIUM: Low (563 mg)
Exchanges: ¾ Meat (extra lean), 4¼ Bread, ¼ Fat

ITALIAN FIRE ROASTED TOMATOES

Slow roasted Roma tomatoes marinated in balsamic vinegar, olive oil, basil and roasted garlic. Approx. 12 oz serving.

✓✓ CALORIES: Very Low (93)   ✓✓ CHOLESTEROL: None (0 mg)
✓✓ FAT: Very Low* (2 g)   SODIUM: Moderate (745 mg)
Exchanges: 3 Veg, ¼ Fat

FAT-FREE RICE PUDDING

Traditional rice pudding with all natural ingredients, but no fat! Approx. 12 oz serving.

✓✓ CALORIES: Very Low (348)   ✓✓ CHOLESTEROL: Very Low (2 mg)
✓✓ FAT: Very Low* (<1 g)   ✓✓ SODIUM: Very Low (71 mg)
Exchanges: 4½ Bread, ¼ Fruit, ½ Milk

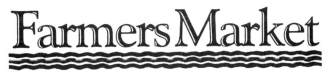

Farmers Market

The finest quality in produce, meat, seafood and gourmet grocery items featuring a unique blend of various food services, including: catering, creative gift baskets, delicacy salads, and in Atrium Court, a garden fresh salad bar and potato bar, wine bar and juice bar for a fast healthy meal. Look for the Chef's Reserve symbol which designates quality products made on the premises. $

Farmers Market

Atrium Court 401 Newport Ctr Dr, Newport Beach, CA 92660   (714) 760-0403
Marbella Plaza 31109 Rancho Viejo Rd, San Juan Capistrano, CA 92675   (714) 248-0838
Lake Mission Viejo 27742 Vista del Lago, Mission Viejo, CA 92692   Opening 1996

ORANGE ROUGHY WRAPPED SALMON
Fresh orange roughy filet wrapped around salmon medallions and poached in a white wine-shallot broth. 10 oz serving.
✓✓ CALORIES: Very Low (295)   ✓ CHOLESTEROL: Low (85 mg)
✓✓ FAT: Very Low* (7 g)   ✓ SODIUM: Low (355 mg)
Exchanges: 4½ Meat, ¼ Veg

BOWTIE PASTA WITH SUNDRIED TOMATO
10 oz serving.
✓ CALORIES: Low (534)   ✓✓ CHOLESTEROL: None (0 mg)
✓✓ FAT: Very Low* (9 g)   ✓✓ SODIUM: Very Low (264 mg)
Exchanges: 4¼ Bread, 1¼ Fat

CHICKEN PRIMAVERA
10 oz breast of chicken stuffed with herbed julienne vegetables and garlic, then baked to perfection in white wine.
✓ CALORIES: Low (467)   CHOLESTEROL: Moderate (221 mg)
✓✓ FAT: Very Low (10 g)   ✓✓ SODIUM: Very Low (231 mg)
Exchanges: 11½ Meat, ½ Veg

TABOULE SALAD
An old world recipe of parsley, tomatoes, cracked wheat mixed with secret herbs & spices for a tasty & healthy salad. 8 oz serving.
✓ CALORIES: Low (370)   ✓✓ CHOLESTEROL: None (0 mg)
✓ FAT: Low* (16 g)   SODIUM: Moderate (740 mg)
Exchanges: 1½ Bread, ¾ Veg, 1½ Fat

GARDEN LENTIL SALAD
Lentils, tomatoes, parsley, lemon and olive oil create a fresh, naturally delicious salad. 8 oz serving.
✓ CALORIES: Low (481)   ✓✓ CHOLESTEROL: None (0 mg)
FAT: Moderate* (22 g)   ✓ SODIUM: Low (447 mg)
Exchanges: 1¾ Bread, ¼ Veg, 2¼ Fat

* Primarily unsaturated fat   *Healthy Dining in Orange County*   **131**

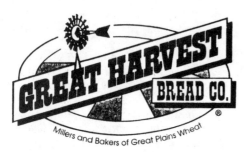

Voted "Best Loaf of Bread" by the Orange County Business Journal, the Great Harvest Bread Co. draws thousands of local residents with its delicious aroma of baking breads. The bread is made the way you would if you had the time -- milling whole wheat flour at the crack of dawn, using no added fats or anything artificial, and hand kneading each loaf. Come in for a sample of the best-tasting, freshest bread anywhere! $

Great Harvest Bread Co.

3972 Barranca Pkwy, Su F1 (Crossroads Shopping Ctr.), Irvine, CA 92714　(714) 552-5442
27261-G La Paz Road, Laguna Niguel, CA 92656　(714) 360-9190

---

9 GRAIN WHOLE WHEAT BREAD†
A moist, hearty bread, filled with a mix of whole wheat, barley, corn, flax, millet, oats, rice, rye and triticale. Perfect for the health-conscious.

✓✓　CALORIES: Very Low (106)　　✓✓　CHOLESTEROL: None (0 mg)
✓✓　FAT: Very Low* (½ g)　　　　　SODIUM: Moderate (245 mg)
Exchanges: 1½ Bread

HONEY WHOLE WHEAT BREAD†
Our most popular whole wheat bread, sweetened with a generous portion of pure northern California honey. Great for sandwiches.

✓✓　CALORIES: Very Low (105)　　✓✓　CHOLESTEROL: None (0 mg)
✓✓　FAT: Very Low* (½ g)　　　　　SODIUM: Moderate (270 mg)
Exchanges: 1½ Bread

OREGON HERB (ONION DILL RYE) BREAD†
Bursting with flavor, this rye bread compliments any meal and makes truly exceptional deli style sandwiches. A favorite with our customers.

✓✓　CALORIES: Very Low (110)　　✓✓　CHOLESTEROL: None (0 mg)
✓✓　FAT: Very Low* (½ g)　　　　　SODIUM: Moderate (243 mg)
Exchanges: 1½ Bread

CINNAMON RAISIN WALNUT WHOLE WHEAT BREAD†
Irresistible! The plump California raisins and walnuts make this a great bread for breakfast, snacks or a meal in itself.

✓　CALORIES: Low (119)　　　　✓✓　CHOLESTEROL: None (0 mg)
✓✓　FAT: Very Low* (2 g)　　　　　SODIUM: Moderate (251 mg)
Exchanges: 1½ Bread

COUNTRY WHITE†
A moist, robust bread, ideal for sandwiches, French toast, or just plain snacking. Made with unbleached flour and pure northern California honey.

✓✓　CALORIES: Very Low (105)　　✓✓　CHOLESTEROL: None (0 mg)
✓✓　FAT: Very Low* (¼ g)　　　　　SODIUM: Moderate (408 mg)
Exchanges: 1½ Bread

CRANBERRY WHITE†
One of our many delicious specialty breads.

✓✓　CALORIES: Very Low (113)　　✓✓　CHOLESTEROL: None (0 mg)
✓✓　FAT: Very Low* (¼ g)　　　　　SODIUM: Moderate (349 mg)
Exchanges: 1½ Bread

Nutrition information supplied by Great Harvest Bread Co., per 50 g serving (approx. 1 slice).

† Side dish guidelines are 1/3 of entree guidelines
✓ Low　✓✓ Very Low

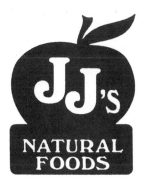

At JJ's Cafe and Juice Bar we use only the finest ingredients when preparing our menu items. Our salad, soups and entrees are made fresh daily right on the premises! All sandwiches and juices are made to order, to give you the freshness and quality you deserve. You can trust JJ's ..... naturally! $

JJ's Natural Foods

18611 Yorba Linda Blvd., Yorba Linda, CA 92686   (714) 777-0845

VEGETARIAN LASAGNA

with spinach, onions, herbs & spices, tofu, low-fat ricotta cheese, marinara sauce, and Jack or Mozzarella cheese topping. (8 oz serving)

✓✓ CALORIES: Very Low (256)   ✓✓ CHOLESTEROL: Very Low (41 mg)
✓✓ FAT: Very Low (10 g)   ✓ SODIUM: Low (466 mg)

Exchanges: ¾ Meat, 1¾ Bread, 1¼ Veg, 1¼ Fat

PEKING BROCCOLI† *(4 oz)*

Organic raw broccoli with bell pepper, sesame seeds, rice vinegar, organic tamari, honey and chili flakes.

✓✓ CALORIES: Very Low (58)   ✓✓ CHOLESTEROL: None (0 mg)
✓✓ FAT: Very Low (1 g)   SODIUM: Moderate (295 mg)

Exchanges: ½ Veg

MARINATED VEGETABLES† *(4 oz)*

Organic raw vegetables with canola oil, lemon juice, balsamic vinegar, oregano, mint, black pepper & salt.

✓✓ CALORIES: Very Low (83)   ✓✓ CHOLESTEROL: None (0 mg)
 ✓ FAT: Low* (6 g)   ✓✓ SODIUM: Very Low (57 mg)

Exchanges: 1 Veg, 1¼ Fat

HERBED OVEN ROASTED POTATOES† *(4 oz)*

Organic red potatoes with olive oil, Italian seasoning, salt & garlic.

 ✓ CALORIES: Low (132)   ✓✓ CHOLESTEROL: None (0 mg)
 ✓ FAT: Low* (4 g)   ✓✓ SODIUM: Very Low (88 mg)

Exchanges: 1¼ Bread, ¾ Fat

---

* Primarily unsaturated fat

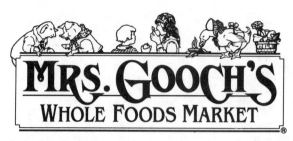

Mrs. Gooch's Whole Foods Market is dedicated to supplying the finest, most natural, wholesome foods available, including an ever-increasing selection of organically grown produce and products with organically grown ingredients. Our savory salads, delectable dressings, steamy soups, enticing entrees and many of our delicious baked goods are prepared in our own kitchen, using time honored recipes with no artificial flavors, artificial colors, artificial sweeteners or preservatives. $

Mrs. Gooch's Whole Foods Markets
14945 Holt Ave, Tustin, CA 92680   (714) 731-3400

TUSTIN CHICKEN
8 oz serving

✓✓ CALORIES: Very Low (302)   ✓ CHOLESTEROL: Low (78 mg)
✓ FAT: Low (13 g)   ✓✓ SODIUM: Very Low (122 mg)
Exchanges: 4 Meat (extra lean), 1¼ Veg, 2 Fat

ROTISSERIE BARBEQUE CHICKEN BREASTS
8 oz serving with 2 Tbs Sauce.

✓ CALORIES: Low (396)   CHOLESTEROL: Moderate (173 mg)
✓ FAT: Low (11 g)   ✓ SODIUM: Low (450 mg)
Exchanges: 9 Meat (extra lean)

SWEET-N-SOUR TOFU
8 oz serving

✓✓ CALORIES: Very Low (134)   ✓✓ CHOLESTEROL: None (0 mg)
✓✓ FAT: Very Low* (2 g)   SODIUM: Moderate (673 mg)
Exchanges: ¾ Meat, 1 Bread, ¾ Veg, ½ Fruit, 1 Fat

HONEY MUSTARD CHICKEN
8 oz serving

✓ CALORIES: Low (367)   ✓ CHOLESTEROL: Low (86 mg)
✓ FAT: Low (12 g)   SODIUM: Moderate (710 mg)
Exchanges: 4 Meat (extra lean), ¼ Veg, 1 Fat

VEGAN POTATO DILL SAUCE WITH TEMPEH
6 oz serving

✓✓ CALORIES: Very Low (217)   ✓✓ CHOLESTEROL: Very Low (14 mg)
✓✓ FAT: Very Low* (8 g)   ✓✓ SODIUM: Very Low (211 mg)
Exchanges: 2 Meat, 1¼ Bread, ¼ Veg, ½ Fat

† Side dish guidelines are 1/3 of entree guidelines

✓ Low   ✓✓ Very Low

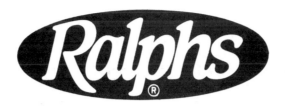

Ralphs Chef Express is pleased to provide nutrition information for those entrees, salads, and side dishes which serve as healthy, delicious choices for consumers concerned with their intake of calories, fat, cholesterol and/or sodium. Chef Express offers the highest quality foods available, at reasonable prices. All menu items are made fresh daily without preservatives, artificial ingredients or MSG. Chef Express departments are not available at all Ralphs stores. For locations contact store management. Not all items available at all times. $

Ralphs -- with 62 Chef Express service deli locations in Orange County.

GRILLED SALMON WITH CHILE CILANTRO MAYONNAISE *(6 oz serving)*
✓✓ CALORIES: Very Low (264)   ✓ CHOLESTEROL: Low (91 mg)
 ✓ FAT: Low* (11 g)   ✓ SODIUM: Low (342 mg)

GARLIC ROASTED CHICKEN# *(6 oz serving)*
✓✓ CALORIES: Very Low (197)   ✓✓ CHOLESTEROL: Very Low (83 mg)
✓✓ FAT: Very Low (7 g)   ✓✓ SODIUM: Very Low (70 mg)

VEGETARIAN LASAGNA# *(6 oz serving)*
✓✓ CALORIES: Very Low (199)   ✓✓ CHOLESTEROL: Very Low (42 mg)
✓✓ FAT: Very Low (5 g)   ✓ SODIUM: Low (416 mg)

SPICY MEXICAN CHICKEN SALAD# *(6 oz serving)*
✓✓ CALORIES: Very Low (209)   ✓✓ CHOLESTEROL: Very Low (42 mg)
 ✓ FAT: Low (11 g)   ✓✓ SODIUM: Very Low (140 mg)

FETTUCCINI WITH VEGETABLES†# *(4 oz serving)*
✓✓ CALORIES: Very Low (107)   ✓✓ CHOLESTEROL: None (0 mg)
 ✓ FAT: Low (5 g)   ✓ SODIUM: Low (104 mg)

FRESH FRUIT SALAD†# *(4 oz serving)*
✓✓ CALORIES: Very Low (96)   ✓✓ CHOLESTEROL: None (0 mg)
✓✓ FAT: None (0 g)   ✓✓ SODIUM: Very Low (9 mg)

CUCUMBER ONION SALAD† *(4 oz serving)*
✓✓ CALORIES: Very Low (40)   ✓✓ CHOLESTEROL: Very Low (<1 mg)
✓✓ FAT: Very Low* (<1 g)   ✓ SODIUM: Low (199 mg)

CARROT AND CELERY SLAW† *(4 oz serving)*
✓✓ CALORIES: Very Low (50)   ✓✓ CHOLESTEROL: Very Low (<1 mg)
✓✓ FAT: Very Low* (<1 g)   SODIUM: Moderate (273 mg)

#Nutrition information supplied by Ralphs Grocery.

* Primarily unsaturated fat
** If you request no added salt

Other

Healthy Dining

Books

Healthy Dining books are also available for the Los Angeles area and the San Diego area. See listings on the next 2 pages for restaurants participating in *Healthy Dining in Los Angeles* and *Healthy Dining in San Diego*.

Healthy Dining in _Los Angeles_

Participating restaurants:

Acapulco
Andree's Oven & Catering
BeauRivage
Bistro 45
Bombay Cafe
Border Grill
Bravo Cucina
Bristol Farms
Bristol's Cafe
Ca'Brea
Cafe La Bohème
Cafe Nordstrom
Carrows
Chasen's
Chin Chin
Chommanade
Clearwater Cafe
Coogie's Beach Cafe
Cutters
Dante's Italian Cuisine
Da Pasquale
DC3
Drago
Earth, Wind & Flour
Edward's Steak House
El Cholo Mexican Restaurant
El Pollo Loco
The Firehouse
Four Seasons Hotel - Gardens Rest.
Fourth Street Grille
   - Guest Quarters Suite Hotel
Gaucho Grill
Granita
Gratis
Green Street
Hugo's
i Cugini Trattoria
Il Cielo
Il Fornaio Cucina Italiana
Il Forno
il Moro
il Pastaio
Inn of the Seventh Ray
Italy's Little
Jack in the Box
Jimmy's
Jimmy's Fish & Grill

JW Marriott Hotel at Century City
Kate Mantilini
Kelly's
Koo Koo Roo
La Frite Cafe
La Luna Ristorante
La Salsa
La Vecchia Cucina
Lido di Manhattan Beach
Louise's Trattoria
Lunaria Restaurant and Jazz Club
Maple Drive
Marix Tex Mex
McCormick & Schmick's
Mi Piace
Michael's
Monroe's of Malibu
Mrs. Gooch's Whole Foods Market
Mum's
Orleans
Papa Jon's
Patina
Piazza Rodeo
Pine Avenue Fish House
Pinot Bistro
Ralphs Grocery
Roxxi
Ruby's Diner
Sabor
Sand Castle
Schatzi on Main
Shenandoah Cafe
Shioji Japanese Restaurant & Sushi Bar
    - Sheraton Long Beach Hotel
Sisley Italian Kitchen
Sizzler
Spago
Taverna Tony Greek Eats and Sweets
Tower Restaurant
Twin Palms
The Warehouse
Water Grill
Wok Spirit
World Cafe
Yangtze
Zach's Italian Cafe
Zenzero

Healthy Dining in San Diego

Participating restaurants:

Anthony's
Bali Hai
Blue Crab
Bully's
Cafe 6TH & K - Clarion Hotel Bay View
Cafe California - at the Broadway
Cafe Greentree
Cafe India
Cafe Nordstrom
Cafe on Park
Cafe Pacifica
Cafe San Diego - Doubletree Hotel
Carmel Highland Doubletree - Terraces Cafe
Carrows
Casa de Bandini
Casa de Pico
Casady's Whole Foods
Chang Cuisine of China
ChickeNest
Chilango's Mexico City Grill
Chili's
Clarion Hotel Bay View - Cafe 6TH & K
COCO'S
CrazyBurro
Croce's
Daily's
Daniel's Market
DiMille's
D'Lish
Doubletree - Cafe San Diego
The Eggery
El Indio
El Pollo Loco
Fifth & Hawthorne
Fish Merchant
French Gourmet
French Pastry Shop
Gentleman's Choice
Great Harvest Bread Co.
Hungry Hunter
Il Fornaio
Ingrid's Wild West Cafe
Jack in the Box
Jimbo's.....Naturally!

KC's Tandoor
Kabul West
Kirby's Cafe
Kung Food Vegetarian Restaurant
La Gran Tapa
La Salsa
Le Meridien Hotel - L'Escale Restaurant
Lino's
Los Cabos
Marina Sea Grill - San Diego Marriott
Montanas American Grill
Mucho Gusto
Nicolosi's
Pacifica Del Mar
Panda Panda
Papachinos
Pasta Experience
Peking Wok
Pick Up Stix
Pizza Nova
Pizzeria Uno
Poseidon
Rainwater's
Ralphs Grocery Chef Express
Rancho el Nopal
Rancho Valencia Resort Restaurant
Royal Thai Cuisine
Ruby's Diner
Salmon House
SandCrab Cafe
Second Nature Vegetarian Cafe
Sheik Cafe
Sheraton Grande Torrey Pines - Torreyana Grill
Sizzler
St. Germain's Cafe
Star of India
T.D. Hays
Terraces Cafe - Carmel Highland Doubletree
T.G.I. Friday's
Thai Chada
Tom Ham's Lighthouse
Torreyana Grill - Sheraton Grande Torrey Pines
Welk Resort Center Restaurant
Wendy's

Each edition has over $200 worth of coupons; $14.95.
To order, see page 144, or call (619) 453-3814 or 1-800-953-DINE

Questionnaire

and Order Form

$3.00 OFF
your next purchase of *Healthy Dining*

We want to know more about you and your thoughts about *Healthy Dining*. So we'll give you $3.00 off your next copy of *Healthy Dining* if you'll return this questionnaire (information is confidential). To thank you, we will contact you when new editions are published and offer $3.00 off the retail price. You may also order now at the discount price (see reverse side).

1. How did you learn about *Healthy Dining in Orange County*?
   ____ Newspaper   ____ Family or friend   ____ Dietitian
   ____ Radio   ____ Restaurant   ____ Personal Trainer
   ____ Television   ____ Health Organization   ____ Fitness Center
   ____ Store _____ ____ Physician   ____ Other _____

2. Are you on any of these special diets?
   ____ weight loss   ____ low-cholesterol   ____ diabetic   ____ vegetarian
   ____ low-fat   ____ low-sodium   ____ general health-conscious

3. Please rate the following features of the book:

	Very helpful	Moderately helpful	Not needed
Chapters on general nutrition	____	____	____
List of restaurants offering healthier items	____	____	____
Specific menu items available at these restaurants	____	____	____
Numerical values of fat, calories, cholesterol, etc.	____	____	____
Categories for "✓ low" and "✓✓ very low"	____	____	____
Restaurant coupons	____	____	____

4. Please list your favorite restaurants from this book:

5. What other restaurants would you like to see in the next edition?

6. What other food or health-related publications do you read? (American Health Magazine, Berkeley Wellness, Nutrition Action Healthletter, Eating Well, Cooking Light, etc.)

7. On average, how many times <u>per month</u> do you dine out? _____

8. Is this book primarily used by: ___ female ___ male ___ both

9. What is the age of the primary user of this book?
   ____ Under 30   ____ 30 to 45   ____ 45 to 60   ____ over 60

10. Would you or any of your personal contacts like more information about: ____ fundraising ____ seminars or community events ____ wholesale prices for *Healthy Dining*?

Other Comments?

OC3

Please complete name and address on reverse side, fold and mail. Photocopy acceptable.   **143**

Fold on lines with address on outside.

Name _____

Address _____

_____

Stamp

Hill & Hill Publishing
P. O. Box 927215
San Diego, CA 92192-7215

Special $3.00 OFF any *Healthy Dining* books.

Order as many as you want at the special discount! It's our thank-you for answering our questionnaire.
You will also receive the $3.00 discount on future editions. Orders normally processed within 1 week.

Quantity			Price
_____	*Healthy Dining in Orange County*	$14.95 - $3.00 discount = $11.95	_____
_____	*Healthy Dining in Los Angeles*	$14.95 - $3.00 discount = $11.95	_____
_____	*Healthy Dining in San Diego*	$14.95 - $3.00 discount = $11.95	_____
		Subtotal	_____
		Tax (7¾% in Orange County)	_____
		Postage ($1.25 for 1st book + 50¢ each for additional books)	_____
		Total	_____

____ Check enclosed   Phone (   ) _____

____ VISA/Mastercard # _____ exp._____ Signature _____

Please fill out questionnaire on reverse and your name & address above. If sending check, make to
Hill & Hill Publishing and fasten your check securely to this sheet or use a separate envelope. Thanks.

Coupons

20% OFF
Entire Meal

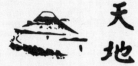

Amachi
Japanese Restaurant

2675 Irvine Ave.
Costa Mesa, CA
(714) 645-5518

Alcoholic beverages excluded.
Up to 4 in party. Not valid with any other offer.

20% OFF
Entire Meal

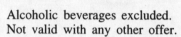

Amelia's

311 Marine Ave, Balboa Island
Newport Beach, CA 92662
(714) 673-6580

Alcoholic beverages excluded.
Not valid with any other offer.

50% OFF
Second Entree

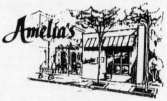

Brazilian
Tropical Cafe

Up to 4 in party.
Not valid with any other offer.

401 Newport Ctr. Dr. #A-106
Newport Beach, CA 720-1522

20% OFF
Entire Meal

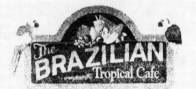

Bukhara
Cuisine of India

7594 Edinger Ave, Huntington Beach
(714) 842-3171
16260 Ventura Blvd #130, Encino
(818) 906-8472

Not valid with any other offer.

20% OFF
Entire Meal

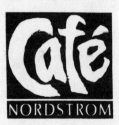

Cafe
Nordstrom

Up to 4 in party.
Alcoholic beverages excluded.
Not valid with any other offer.

South Coast Plaza, Brea Mall,
Main Place (Santa Ana), Montclair,
& Tyler Mall (Riverside)

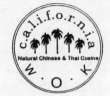
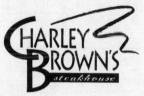

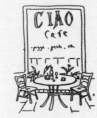

Free Entree

With purchase of one entree
of equal or greater value,
any weekday.
Not valid with any other special offers.

Ciao

223 Marine Avenue
Balboa Island, CA 92662
(714) 675-4070

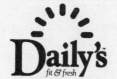

$1.00 OFF

**any sandwich,
salad, or entree.**
One coupon per customer.
Not valid with any other offer.

Daily's
fit & fresh

Tustin: 498 E. First Street
Laguna Niguel: 27000 Alicia Parkway

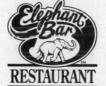

20% OFF
Food Check

Up to 8 in party.
Not valid with alcoholic beverages or desserts.
Not valid with any other offer.

Elephant Bar

14303 Firestone Blvd, La Mirada
25250 East La Paz Road, Laguna Hills

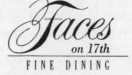

20% OFF
Entire Meal

Alcoholic beverages excluded.
Up to 4 in party. Not valid with other offers or coupons.

Faces
on 17th

1615 East 17th Street
Santa Ana 972-2200

Free Meal

**With purchase of one meal
of equal or greater value.**

Not valid with any other special offers.

Ferdussi
Taste of Persia

3605 S. Bristol Street, Santa Ana
(corner of Bristol & MacArthur, one block
north of South Coast Plaza)   545-9096

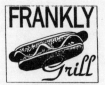
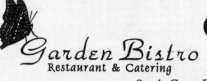
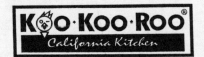

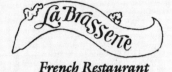
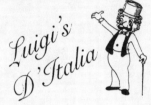
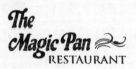

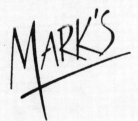

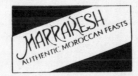
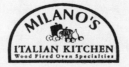
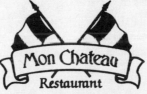
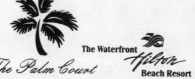

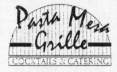
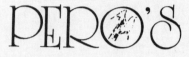
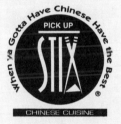
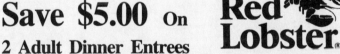
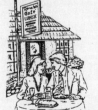

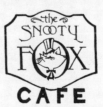

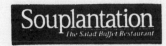
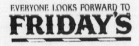
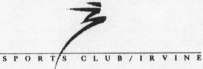
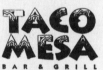

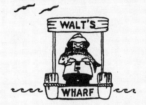
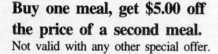

Fast Food

Free BBQ Chicken Sandwich

Carl's Jr.®

when you purchase any Charbroiled Chicken Sandwich at regular price after 4 pm.
One coupon per customer per visit. One discount per coupon.
Not valid with any other offer or discount. Tax not included.
Present this coupon when ordering.

Offer valid through
Dec. 31, 1997 at any participating
Orange County Carl's Jr.® Restaurant

©1995 Carl Karcher Enterprises, Inc.

Coupon   *Healthy Dining in Orange County*   Coupon

$1.00 OFF

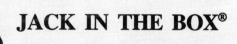

JACK IN THE BOX®

Chicken Teriyaki Bowl

Only 1.5 grams of fat!
Served after 10:30 am. Please present coupon when ordering.
One coupon per customer. One offer per coupon.
Not valid in combination with any other offer.

Valid through 12/31/97
at all participating
JACK IN THE BOX® Restaurants
Line #269

Coupon   *Healthy Dining in Orange County*   Coupon

Free Sandwich

Wendy's

With purchase of one sandwich
of equal or greater value.
Please present coupon when ordering.

Valid at Orange County Wendy's
Not valid with other special offers.

Markets, Delis
and Bakery

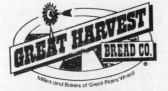

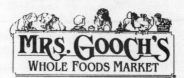

Index

Index by Cuisine

Index by Location

Index by Location (continued)

Index by Location (continued)

Index by Location (continued)

Alphabetical Index